How Am I Doing?

40 Conversations to Have with Yourself

Dr. Corey Yeager

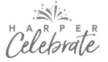
HARPER
Celebrate

How Am I Doing?

Published by Harper Celebrate, an imprint of HarperCollins Focus LLC.

Any internet addresses (websites, blogs, etc.) in this book are offered as a resource. They are not intended in any way to be or imply an endorsement by HarperCollins Focus LLC, nor does HarperCollins Focus LLC vouch for the content of these sites for the life of this book.

ISBN 978-1-4002-5105-6 (TP)
ISBN 978-1-4002-3679-4 (Audiobook)
ISBN 978-1-4002-3678-7 (epub)
ISBN 978-1-4002-3676-3 (HC)

Printed in Malaysia

25 26 27 28 29 VPM 5 4 3 2 1

Contents

CONTENTS

Foreword

As I write this foreword, I've just wrapped up practice, and I'm preparing for a weekend on the road to play for the Detroit Pistons, barely unpacking from the last trip. In between games and practice and plane flights and working with coaches and connecting with staff, at the end of the day, my job doesn't end at the sound of a buzzer. When I leave work, I go back to my favorite job—being a dad to my three-year-old little girl. It's a lot to manage, but I can't imagine anything more important.

I'm on a journey to find out how great I can be, and what I'm finding is that with every new opportunity, there's greater responsibility. My main responsibility on and off the court is to elevate my game as well as those around me. People are counting on me, and they should, because being a leader makes me who I am.

Greatness isn't just going to happen. Greatness comes from preparation, and it starts with coming into awareness of what's important to me and creating a plan of how I'm going to achieve that. Greatness means taking time to block out what everyone else wants for me and instead focus on who I want to be.

One of my favorite places to focus is sitting courtside with O.G. Dr. Corey Yeager. He's technically a life coach and advisor, but to me, he's more like an uncle. The thing I can count on when I take that seat beside Doc is he never wants anything *from* me but instead wants everything *for* me. I can ask him anything, and if he can help, he will. It never feels like he's trying to analyze me or diagnose what he's observed in me. He's just an uncle who just so happens to have a psychological framework. My relationship with the doc over the last year has shown me that talking about mental wellness doesn't have to be sterile. It can be a conversation. These conversations don't have to be a big deal. They can happen anywhere you need them to happen.

That's what you're going to find in this book, *How Am I Doing?* It's a selection of forty fluid conversations to better get to know who you are, what you want, and where you're headed. As Dr. Yeager opens up about his life in the pages of this book, you have the opportunity to open up about your story, too. And let me tell you, I've never regretted a conversation with Doc. These questions are your shot to get to define your own path toward greatness, whatever that may be, and take ownership of who you're becoming.

I'm known for my career in the NBA, but the thing you may

not know is that becoming a great dad is equally as important to me. My daughter is my whole world, and I love her more than I can express. I know I need to become the best dad I can be because she's counting on me. The work Doc and I do is just as much about my personal life as it is about my professional one. The two intersect, and he understands that pursuing happiness, intentionality, and excellence can't be compartmentalized.

The interesting thing the Doc pointed out to me is that who I am in one space impacts who I am in another. One thing we have discussed is the importance of my basketball family as well as my family of origin. My family's presence in the stands puts me in the right mental space, and I perform better knowing I have them on my team. It might just feel like a nice story at first, but bringing this into awareness actually reveals something deeper than that—the core to what makes me *me*, and what greatness might mean for me on and off the court. This kind of personal and professional awareness makes me a better person in all the spaces I move through.

In this book, the Doc talks a lot about awareness, and how awareness is the first step to unlocking who you are. Something we talk about at the Pistons is this idea of *restoration*—that the greatest version of our team already exists; we just have to find the blueprint to restore it back to its original form. Similarly, this book is about restoration of yourself. It's not going to tell you how you need to change your life or give you a clear plan of what you need to do next. What it will give you is the awareness you need to take the next steps to restore yourself and step into the greatest version of you.

This is a journey of awareness and empowerment you won't regret, and it all starts with one simple question: *How are you doing?*

Cade Cunningham
Detroit Pistons, NBA

Introduction

To me, therapy is conversation. And conversation—when there's humor, openness, and curiosity—is like playing on a playground. We take turns. We tell stories. And neither of us knows what we'll discover.

I came to psychotherapy after nearly two decades living my dream of playing pro football. I made it pretty far but didn't get all the way to the NFL—which meant I was free to find a new field of play in therapy. It took a lot of work to get here, but at the end of the day, it doesn't feel like work.

At therapy's core, we're talking. And I love talking. Just like with football, I don't always have to have the right answer. It's okay for me to stumble. It's okay for you to stumble. Because sometimes we stumble into magic.

Four years ago, I transitioned from working as a therapist in the Minneapolis public schools—a role I still treasure—to providing sports-based therapy to professional athletes. My clients and office spaces have changed, but ultimately, I'm still just having conversations. These days my office is at the Pistons Performance Center (PPC), where the Detroit Pistons practice. I don't wear a suit, and I don't approach anyone from on high. I just show up and show them I'm present. The players know they can call me anytime day or night. And sometimes they do.

You'll often hear me chatting with the players. "How you livin'? You good?" I say as a player approaches me on the bench. "Come holla at me over here."

Or I'll give them a simple, "How you doin'?"

This book puts that one simple question in *your* court. I break down the larger question, "How am I doing?" into forty smaller questions to help you answer that big one. Your number one goal as you read should be to cultivate a better sense of awareness—becoming curious of who you are and how you got where you are. Only then you can start intentionally making better choices for who you want to be.

Everyone has thoughts and feelings going on under the surface, underneath their awareness. In therapy we call this the subconscious. I like to describe consciousness as the front stage—this is where you see the actors performing. The subconscious is the backstage—all the costumes and scenery changes that you don't see. I want you to tap into what's going on backstage, in your subconscious.

You'll also hear me talk about roots a lot. We are not going to stay on the surface here. We're going to ask a lot of deep questions—questions inside of other questions—and we'll keep going until we find answers.

We're not seeking behavior modification in these pages. I practice narrative-solution focused therapy. That means I dig into a space and get content-laden stories. I think of narrative-solution focused therapy like this. Imagine you're going to have a backyard party, but the yard is covered with dandelions. It looks like you don't spend any time taking care of it. So, you mow. The lawn looks great, and you appear to have it all together. But four days later the dandelions are back. Why? Because you didn't do anything to impact the root system.

In narrative therapy, we're not going to mow. We're going way underneath the surface. Our hands will be covered in dirt. We're going to spend the whole afternoon out there pulling up the entire root system. If we can get to the root, we can better fix the issue for the long term. It's a longer, messier, and more frustrating process.

Throughout this book you'll be pulling up those dandelions. I'll be asking you to recall specific moments, because your content-laden stories are the cornerstone to entering your world. So go ahead and get your notes app open or grab a journal, or maybe you want to walk and talk into your phone. Whatever feels most comfortable for you.

The therapeutic playground sounds like a fun place, but it has its raised voices, hurt feelings, and tears, just like a real playground. It's not always a serene place. Sometimes you will have to fight for resolution. You'll have to be open to the change and growth these battles usher in. My task as a therapist is to be present. That's your task as a reader here too. Be present for yourself. Show up for these questions. Reflect on them. Bring your own thoughts and your own questions.

While I can't be there to hold your story the way I would in person, I'm going to do my best to walk this journey with you. I'll tell you about my struggles and my experience. I'll ask you to stay engaged and work hard. I'll give you prompts and activities to engage with on the page and in the mirror. This deep heart-work and the pages you write will be a vessel for your story. Who knows? Together we might stumble into magic.

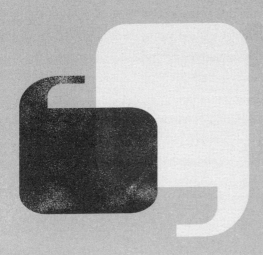

It's okay for me to stumble.
It's okay for you to stumble.
Because sometimes we stumble
into magic.

Who is the most important person in your life?

When you think of the most important person in your life, you might think of one of the people you've committed your life to. Maybe your spouse or a child or a longtime friend. You may think of a parent or grandparent who sacrificed so much to help you grow into who you are today. Or maybe you think of one of the loyal, hardworking people who depend on you at work.

But if a family member, friend, or colleague is the most important person in your life, and everything you do is for them, then where do *you* come in? Are you the *second* most important person? Third, fourth, fifth in line?

You may not realize it, but *you* are the most important person in your life. While you might think prioritizing yourself is selfish or arrogant, I hope to convince you it's not. In fact, it's essential to your well-being and foundational to every other question in this book. Facing up to challenges, becoming intentional with your day, making better decisions, improving relationships—you can't tackle any of those goals until you recognize the position *you're* here to play.

Even though I'm a generous guy and I'm happy to share what I have, I still recognize myself as the top dog in my world. And that means sometimes I have to be generous to myself, give myself the same time and attention and grace I give others. Before I can be a good brother, father, husband, friend, therapist, or coach to anyone, I have to be a good Corey for Corey. When it's my turn to take the shot, I take it. When it's my turn to step up to bat, I step up. When opportunities come to put myself first for my own well-being, I take responsibility for my own needs.

Here's an example. When I'm starting to feel overwhelmed, I tell my wife, Carrie, that I'm taking a Corey day. That means I won't be fielding any calls, even from her. I've learned to make this preemptive move before I become submerged and start making poor decisions. I won't be able to take care of someone else who is overwhelmed when I'm in the same space myself.

This is what I mean by putting myself first. It doesn't mean I don't want to help others. Being of service to others is vital to me. As you'll see in the pages ahead, it's central to my identity. But I am aware of where I need to be mentally to be able to serve others. On days when the gas tank is on empty, I need to fill it up before I go anywhere or do anything. There are afternoons I literally sit in a chair in my living room and refuse to answer the door when people ring the doorbell. If they peer inside the house, they can even see me sitting there. That's how comfortable I have become with putting myself first in this context.

I want to help you put yourself first too.

To be clear, this is not carte blanche to do whatever the heck you want. There will be situations when you're not the priority, and it isn't really about you. Putting someone else's needs first can be the appropriate action in many situations. Staying up late to help your child with her homework, or giving up your seat on the subway to someone who needs it, doesn't mean you're not the most important person. Your role in these situations is to be the adult or to be the good citizen. The difference is you're moving consciously, not reflexively. You're moving with awareness.

As you move through this book, I will be gently prompting you to put yourself first. Along the way I want you to notice when and where you hesitate. Keep asking questions. I don't expect things to change overnight here or anywhere else, but gaining more awareness of where you fall on your list of priorities is the very first step.

TELL YOUR STORY

So let me ask you again: Who is the most important person in your life? (I hope you answered "I am.") How does embracing your role as the star in your own life make you feel?

When you're getting overwhelmed, take a moment to pause and make a plan to protect yourself. Can you say no to an upcoming plan? Can you let the phone go to voicemail? What are some other ways you can put yourself and your needs first?

Keep a log in your calendar or notes app for the next few days. Make two columns. On one side, list the occasions when you put yourself first. On the other, list the moments when you hesitate. Notice examples of each throughout your day. At the end of the week, circle back. Consider imbalances and ask yourself, *Where do I need to make a change?*

Consider the last time you felt completely out of balance. Maybe you hit a wall and burned out over a busy schedule. Maybe you just woke up one day and thought, *What's the point of it all?* Go back into that moment and write it down in your journal, as if you were telling a story. Who were you seeking to please? Was it you or someone else?

What are your wildest dreams?

When I began studying psychology, I started dreaming about a career that would connect my experience in pro sports with my newfound passion for therapy. *Sports and therapy? Nah, those two don't belong together. Bring the dream down, Corey. It doesn't have to be so big.* Now I'm in the NBA, which was a wild dream of mine. I didn't even play basketball to get here! But I pursued a passion to become a therapist, got my doctorate, and it ultimately led to my dream job. It's still wild, but my career is a testament to the fact that wild dreams are not out of your reach.

It's important that we keep a wild dream outstretched in front of us. When we have the shape of our dreams, we're able to intentionally organize and prioritize small, daily tasks. I set macro goals—*Where do I need to be five years from now?* And I set micro goals—*What do I need to do today to move toward that goal?* The macro and the micro need to line up. When they don't, well, that's when we feel offtrack.

What is one of your wildest dreams? And when I say wild, I don't mean impossible. I can dream about running the fastest 100 meters ever, but that goes beyond wild and into the impossible. For me, wild was combining two unlikely fields into one career. Now for me to become the fastest man alive—looking at Usain Bolt in the rearview mirror—I'd have to get an upgraded set of lungs. But I knew a lot about both pro sports and psychology. What I didn't know was how they might come together.

It may not always be obvious how to pursue a wild dream. Maybe you're considering what you want out of life, and your desires seem as oppositional as being a Mets fan and a Yankees fan at the same time. It takes a real dreamer to consider how to bring those desires together, but it's not impossible if you know what you're doing. Keep following your passions—in the simple, daily pursuits and in the riskier, bigger moves—and see if that dream starts to become more of a reality. Being the fastest runner on earth? Impossible. Finding an unusual new path? A wild dream within reach.

Step into the playground. *Wildest* means there are no naysayers. *Wildest* means there's no one pointing at the clock saying you don't have enough time. *Wildest* means you dare to imagine what the future can possibly hold. Later you can bring the dream down to an achievable level. Later you set macro goals and micro goals. Later you can ask, *How the hell could I ever achieve that?*

Why not dream wildly? This is a space you get to author! You have to play with that space. You *get to* play with that space. Let your mind run rampant into the beauty of those wild dreams.

TELL YOUR STORY

Take out ten to fifteen index cards. Write a wild dream on each one. Preposterous dreams. Never-in-a-million-years dreams. Remember who you were before the age of twelve when people told you to stop pretending.

Look through your deck of wild dreams. Which one feels the best when you look at it? Post it somewhere you can see it in your house.

How can you take one of those big, broad dreams and make it specific to you? Through this book you'll gain clarity on your values, your sense of humor, your sacred spaces, and your nonnegotiables. Keep looking back at this card, and get *specific* about how you can shape your dream.

Perhaps your dream is to open a coffeehouse. That's a broad and wonderful dream, but it will be *better* if you infuse it with other elements that make you unique. Maybe you value making opportunities for low-income peers in your community, so you source your workers accordingly. Maybe you imagine the space is filled with the scent of pine, because that reminds you of holiday vacations visiting your grandmother. Maybe dogs in funny hats just make you laugh, and so you fill the walls with pictures of weird dogs you've seen around town. What's important here is that you get specific about your dreams, and you make it specific to your passions, your sadness, your happiness, and your most lighthearted self. Don't you want to chase after *that*?

Who knows you best?

My mother is my truth teller. Her advice has carried me throughout my life (she's known me since the moment I arrived!). But if I said my mother knows me best, I'd be overlooking someone very important.

When I ask this question to my clients, their answers are varied. I hear about boyfriends and wives, friends, children, coworkers, aunts, uncles, cousins, teammates, roommates. I'm glad to hear my clients have supportive relationships. Maybe you would answer the same way. I don't doubt any one of these individuals know an enormous amount about you. They might know your pet peeves and your dreams, your favorite foods and the things that make you laugh out loud for no good reason.

But do they know *everything*? Does your mom or husband

or best friend know *every* secret in your life? Everything you've ever thought or done? They couldn't possibly.

Only one person does.

The answer to this question for me—and for all of us—is the same. The only person who really knows all the pieces of you is *you*.

What are the implications of this reframe? It means that when big questions and decisions arise, you probably already have the answers. It's like insider trading—only legal. Think about it. When you ask someone for advice, don't you know the answer you want to hear most of the time? *Should I take this new job or stick with the one I have? Should I study medicine or engineering? Should I move to the East Coast to keep this relationship? Should I stay home with the baby or put her in daycare? Should I ask for a raise?* We often look to others, seeking confirmation of what we already know.

This realization leads to a question: Do you trust yourself? The answer is pretty simple. If you don't, it's likely because you don't have experience. And society hasn't told you to trust yourself. Instead, it's told you that there's always someone out there with all the answers. The expert, the guru, the coach, the author, the professor, the therapist, the guy giving the TED Talk. Instead of trusting yourself, you learn to trust others to be your mirror. That becomes your default.

That's a habit I'd encourage you to change. But you can't just snap your fingers and learn to trust yourself. Trust is built over time. Building this within yourself is critical and takes a hell of a lot of practice. The first step is just realizing that you are the authority on yourself.

I want you to start engaging with yourself more often— asking yourself more questions and listening to the answers before you ask anybody else. You don't have to tackle major life decisions right away. Instead, begin to build that trust with small decisions. Then when you are faced with major life decisions, you've already built the trust muscle. The deep knowledge into the subject matter—you had that the whole time. You just have to learn to trust the real expert. You.

TELL YOUR STORY

Is there someone with more insight into who you are than you possess? Who? What makes you think they have more clarity?

For an upcoming decision, get a read on what you think and feel before you ask others, even those who (almost) know you best. Try writing down your take on the situation. Perhaps you'd like to make a pros/cons list. Do you know what you're hoping to hear?

Now that you've looked inward, turn to a trusted family member, friend, or advisor and ask for input.

Think of a recent decision you made that turned out to be a good one. It can be something small, like bowing out of an unnecessary meeting on a day when you were overbooked. Take a moment to simply celebrate the decision you made and the action you took.

When do you find it easiest to tune into your own voice? In the shower? On a walk? In the moments before you fall asleep or right after you wake up? As you're preparing dinner? Try to become aware of the times when your own thoughts and insights are most accessible.

Who is the author of your life story?

I was a big kid. Strong. People took one look at me and said, "You're going to be a Kansas City Chief." My dad was a huge football fan and had been a running back, and he passed his love of football on to me. So I started playing at age five and played with the same kids all the way through high school. I happened to be good at the sport, not just big, and was eventually recruited to play college ball. I'll be honest, I didn't study during my years at Long Beach State since, in my mind, I was headed for the pros. Besides, hours of training on the field didn't leave much time for *The Iliad* or quantum mechanics. I had my own battles to fight, the velocity of the football to calculate.

I did workouts with the Cowboys and the Los Angeles

Rams. I even signed a contract with a semipro league in South Carolina. I got all the way to the NFL draft, and then, for the first time in my life, I fumbled. I didn't get picked. At the crucial moment in my story, I failed. I was crushed. I was lost. For five years I was in no-man's-land, going from job to job trying to find myself.

But it turns out, all endings are just opportunities for new beginnings.

The end of my football career was just the beginning of a whole new part of my story. The second act included becoming a researcher, a marriage and family therapist, an activist, a life coach for the Detroit Pistons, and now an author. Every job I have today is the result of failure combined with curiosity—a dangerously fantastic combination if you ask me. Not to mention I'm also a husband, a father, a friend, and a student. None of these pieces is the *whole* story but each part adds to it.

We all have a story to write. Too often we allow others to write our story. We follow the plot outline they create for us. *You're going to be a doctor since you're good with your hands. You're never going to settle down. You'd be a great lawyer. You're tall; you must be a basketball player.* We hear what others think our story should be, and we follow the dreams they set for us. Often these messages come from well-intentioned parents and older relatives who are holding on to their unlived dreams.

Our first step here, as in everything we're practicing, is to allow awareness. When I say you need to be the author of your story, I'm not saying you can't receive guidance from others. You have your important people around you (what I call your "supreme court," which we'll get to later) and all kinds of other bright, curious people in your life. Their thoughts and opinions can lead you down new paths and can stretch you to think fresh or dream bigger. But no matter their influence, other people shouldn't *write* your story.

To write your story requires self-reflection. You need to have a sense of who you are and where you're going. What makes you smile? Ask yourself why. What's a memory from childhood that makes you feel alive? Ask yourself why. What scares you about the next five years? Ask yourself why.

This one word, *why*, is the beginning of knowing yourself, and knowing yourself is the beginning of your authorship of your life. Eventually you can exchange that word *why* and start asking *how*. But first seek clarity on what led you to where you are, and soon you can pick up the pen and write from there.

TELL YOUR STORY

Are you the author of your story? If you aren't, who's holding the pen?

When you were young, did people typecast you? What were some of the roles they thought you would play? How do you feel about those roles?

On a page in your journal, draw eight to ten circles. In each circle, write one of your identities—parent, gardener, kayaker, baker, etc. You can also add more abstract identities like adventurer or extrovert. If you think of more than ten, draw more circles. Do all the identities fit who you are and who you want to be? Are there any identities you might want to let go of?

What kind of genre are you writing with your life? Check all that apply (some of them overlap). This exercise should be fun. Don't take it too seriously.

Adventure	Creation myth
Romance	Epic
Thriller	Supernatural
Superhero	Satire
Revenge	Fairy tale

If your life were a movie, what would you title it? What character are you playing? The lead? The sidekick? The villain?

Do you have an encouraging inner voice?

We're playing the Cavaliers. We're down two. The point guard is dribbling the ball. The coach shouts at him to shoot. The guard dribbles the ball off his foot, and it goes out of bounds. The player knows he screwed up. *Everyone* knows he screwed up.

We could ask what happened, how it went so wrong. But here's the more interesting question: What is the player saying in his head? *Oh my god, you're an idiot. That was a disaster. You let everyone down.*

Or are his words gentler? *Yeah, I screwed up, but I'm going to make it up.*

In both scenarios, the action was the same. But the self-talk that followed? Worlds apart.

That's the difference between positive and negative self-talk. Negative self-talk is an endless echo chamber—old criticism bouncing back, new opportunity blocked out. You might experience it in any area of life, not just on the court. Maybe you're on your way to a family holiday, worried about how others will perceive you. *You haven't lost the weight,* you say to yourself, heart rate starting to climb. *You told people you were going on a diet! Now what are they going to think? You're a train wreck.* If someone else spoke to us like this, would we be friends with that person?

Since you're the most important person in your life, it follows that your voice is going to have a powerful influence. Most of us underestimate that power. We have to start tuning in more deeply to that voice. What is yours saying? Is it encouraging? Defeatist? Quick to blame? Quick to make you feel ashamed? The more positive the talk, the more positive your day. It's the difference between a coach who is quick to criticize and point out flaws and one whose words lift you up. The human body has approximately 40 trillion cells.[1] Every time you say something to yourself, positive or negative, you are directing all 40 trillion of those cells to uphold that thought.

Let's switch over to baseball. You're on deck, just getting ready to walk to the batter's box. You imagine the last two times at bat you struck out, leaving players stranded on base. Do you tell yourself, *Wow, you just* keep *screwing up. You have almost no chance of getting a hit*?

Or do you try a different approach? *This is what I do for a living. I got this. Let's go.*

The ball may not soar into the grandstands on your next swing, even with that confident cheerleader whispering inside your head. But I promise you this—it's got a better chance when you're looking up.

In this country we're taught a myth that rugged individualism is the ideal, that we're all responsible for our own wins and losses. I think this connects to our negative self-talk. *It's on you to figure things out. If you're not successful, it's because* you *didn't do what* you *were supposed to.* When we mess up, we're quick to accept blame. But we're starting to discover as a people just how flawed this way of thinking is when not everyone begins in the same place or is treated the same way.

Being a Black man in America, I know I'm going to encounter tons of negative spaces. I'm not going to add to that with my own negative talk. My task is to move with positivity. Even if no one else has it for me, I have it for myself. No matter who you are, there are people lined up to get in your way and become hurdles in your life. You sure as hell don't need to join them. You can change how the conversation goes by starting with how you talk to yourself.

TELL YOUR STORY

Take a few minutes today to listen to your voice. Don't tell your voice what to say—just listen. Is the voice encouraging? Discouraging? Blaming? Hopeful? Pessimistic? Forward-looking? Backward-looking? Anxious? Compassionate?

Why is your voice that way? Did you hear similar voices from people around you growing up? Do you remember when you first started talking to yourself this way? Do you talk like that to other people?

Track your voice over several days, noting the time of day, what you said, and the situation. Whenever you catch negative self-talk, mark down a negative sign or a sad face. When you hear something positive, mark down a positive sign or smiley face.

After you've filled in your self-talk tracker, do you notice any patterns in positivity or negativity at different times? If you notice differences, make a note of the situations where you have positive talk and those where you have negative talk. Are there some situations where you tend to go easier or harder on yourself? Look back at the end of the three days and think about how you might want to change things going forward.

Just for fun, impersonate the most wildly upbeat and enthusiastic coach you can imagine, as if Ted Lasso is whispering in your ear right now. What does he or she say? *You got this. You can't possibly fail. You've been training for this your entire life. You're in control. You're the G.O.A.T. Go get 'em. There's no stopping you now.*

Who is on your supreme court?

When I was recruited by multiple colleges, I received thirty-one Division I football offers from across the country. Kentucky, Florida, Indiana—they all looked like the view from the top of a rollercoaster. My dad had passed away. I didn't have anyone in my life to help me decide which offer to accept. I ended up going to Long Beach State because my sister, Sharon, lived there.

Was Long Beach State the right decision? A few weeks in, I didn't think so. I had come from a rural community in Kansas and now the center on the team was a Jewish guy from New York who didn't believe me when I said I'd never had a bagel and lox. "Come on, dude, you're lying," he said. I was used to the Midwest, where the world was Black and white, literally. I didn't feel like I fit into this mosaic of cultures. (Fast-forward a few decades, I married into a Jewish family and we eat bagels and lox at my house every weekend.) Plus, all my time was taken up with football and hanging out at the bar where we got free Coors Light after practice. I didn't go to class—the coaches changed my failing grades to keep me eligible. Actually, there was one class I did try to show up for—the Exploitation of the Black Athlete. (The irony was lost on me.) Between the beer and the football, I had no time to see my sister, the whole reason I'd chosen the university.

A week into the first semester, I called my mom. "Long Beach might not be the right place for me," I told her, trying to hide the shakiness in my voice. She didn't pull any punches. "You chose it," she told me. "No one forced you. It's time to step up and figure out how to make that choice the right one." In that moment, my own personal supreme court was born. My mother's statement was simple, but it had a major impact on my life trajectory. My problem wasn't about making the right choice. The harder work was making the choice right.

Choosing a college may have been the first big decision in my life, but it was far from my last. Decision points multiplied in the years that followed—whether to move to Minneapolis for a relationship (I did), whether to marry Carrie (I did that, too, though she wasn't the woman who brought me back to the Midwest), whether to have children (check), whether to leave a great union job (I left)—coming at me fast and furious. I knew

I had to stick with decisions I made, but I still needed help making them in the first place. We all do.

Over the years, in all the different decisions I have had to make, I've relied on my supreme court to help me. You can call the group what you will—your team, your cabinet, your posse. Doesn't matter, just make sure you have one. These are the three to five people who you can go to for advice and wisdom on big life decisions. They tell you the truth based on what they know about you and what they've heard you say.

These truth tellers don't need access to some ultimate truth. They just have to be willing to tell the truth as they see it based on what they know about you. We all need people like my mom, people who aren't pulling punches. They don't have to be the people you like the best. One might be a friend you've known since first grade; another could be a coworker you met in your fifties when you had a better idea of who you were and where you wanted to go.

Your truth tellers don't have to agree with your worldview, but they do need to *know* you. In fact, often the best advice a truth teller can give is to remind you to take your own advice. You're not looking for people to let you vent or be your cheer-leading squad. You have friends for that. One of my great joys is when someone challenges me in conversation, which can lead to a broadening and deepening of my own awareness.

Be intentional about selecting your supreme court and be clear about what you want from them. Sometimes you'll have different members you turn to for different topics. You may need someone in your field who knows you in that setting for a specific problem. I have an advisor in my field to whom I turn for anything related to my psychotherapeutic work. You may have a coworker for work decisions, a spiritual leader for faith crossroads, etc. But just like I wouldn't go to my advisor about my personal relationships, each supreme court member will play a different role.

You won't assemble your truth tellers overnight. My court has been developed over many years. And as important as it has been to trust my gut, it's been just as crucial to have folks around me who can repeat my worldview back to me.

Once you have a supreme court assembled, you have a powerful resource. But with every decision, first ask yourself the hard questions. Only then will you be able to talk to the truth tellers. Only then will you be able to hear the truth of what they have to say.

TELL YOUR STORY

Who are your truth tellers? Who can you count on to tell you things you may not want to hear?

How do you feel when someone challenges you in conversation? Start to take note of your reaction. Is it open? Defensive? Do you feel the need to prove yourself? Now step back even further and ask, *Is this the reaction I'd like to have?*

Now consider this—what about when it's your turn to tell the truth to someone else? How can you be a good supreme court member? Ask questions. Get inside your friend's head. Try to understand their values and how they view the world. Curiosity always pushes us into deeper conversations. You have the power to help others move into a space of understanding.

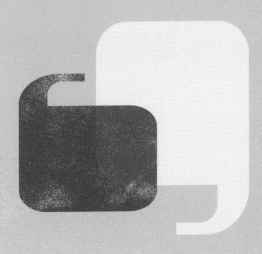

Often the best advice a truth teller can give is to remind you to take your own advice.

Do you allow yourself to imagine what your future could be?

L eading up to a recent interview, I rehearsed the upcoming conversation several times in my head. I knew I didn't need to cram on the content, but I still needed to prepare. My favorite way to do that is to imagine the questions I might get asked and then think through the way I might respond. Before I got to the interview, I'd already envisioned several mini-dramas in my head.

For me, this is play.

As a therapist I like to say, "Get me into the playground of your life." When that person and I are engaged in a symbiotic conversation, we can try on different ideas, assume new identities, use new expressions. It doesn't mean we're changing everything in our real lives any more than a child pretending to be a princess is actually a princess. We're playing. We're reimagining who we *could* be.

Sometimes I almost feel like an acting coach. If someone wants to be more adaptable, we'll visualize an upcoming meeting and imagine all the ways it could go. It's a low-stakes rehearsal. What will it look like? What will the person feel? The next week we'll talk about how the real-life meeting went.

The guys on the basketball team I work with have embraced visualization on the sidelines. I might ask them to visualize what's going to happen in the second half of the game. *If the other team defended this play, what would you do?* Then we rehearse another version, and another. Playing in this directed, imaginative space offers us the opportunity to step into our futures with preparation and flexibility. We don't need to lock in on how the future *needs* to go, just how it *could* go.

Chances are, that next play won't go the way you imagined. But that's okay, because now you've primed yourself with the power of your imagination to be ready to pivot. You've already been there in your mind. You're ready.

In the playground there is opportunity. You can have a more directed type of visualization, like my interview or a specific basketball game. Or you can have something more free-form, where you let the ideas unfold organically, simply trying on different iterations of who you could be.

As a child your imagination was home. Pretend play was

your language. But when you were barely a decade into the world, society started telling you, *You have to start thinking about high school. Your grades are going to count now. Time to buck up.* And from then on the playground folded in on itself like a vortex, leaving in its place a checklist. Life became about accomplishments, career, a steady relationship—always ushering in that next stage of life. You were taught that imagination was something to say goodbye to, like outgrown Nike Shark football cleats.

Stepping back into the playground may require a bit of patience at first. We can't force things to happen there. It has to evolve naturally. This is tough, because a lot of us are used to taking direction, receiving an agenda, and plowing ahead. I'm asking you to sit back.

The playground is an intuitive space. Following your imagination requires trusting what you *sense* to be true, not calculating next steps through external research or data. You'll have to rely on your internal guide here. If you haven't spent a lot of time listening, it will take practice to understand the language they speak. But if you keep showing up to the playground, trust that the childhood version of you will eventually start showing up too. And, paradoxically, that childhood version is the one who will help you imagine the future.

TELL YOUR STORY

Write down five things coming up today or this week that are causing you anxiety or anticipation. Pick one. Then take a few deep, slow breaths and visualize that situation. What images come to mind? Like you're watching a movie in your head, play out how you anticipate that situation could go. Visualize the best movie you can dream of. Now visualize the worst movie you can dream of. Now you know your parameters!

Let's pick a role you want to try on. Do you ever say, "I wish I could be more like [X]"? Who is X, and what are their qualities you admire? Pick one of those qualities, and visualize a version of you assuming that quality. What will it look like to act with that quality? What will it feel like? The more detail you can use to set the scene, the better. Will you be at home? At work? At a neighborhood meeting? Who else will be there? How will they react?

Write out a short script anticipating a conversation that will take place later today. After writing out this script, what are questions you have for yourself? What are ways you might help yourself make the most of this moment?

Iterate and rewrite this scene several more times, and then let it go. Move on to the next task in your day. You're as ready as you're going to be.

What is your genius?

When we think of geniuses, we might think of Albert Einstein, Mozart, or Toni Morrison. Or maybe we heard about the gifted twelve-year-old boy who got accepted into college to study aerospace engineering. These people have an intelligence level way beyond what most of us could ever dream of. But we all still have a genius. We're all NBA players in our own realm.

When I ask most people about their genius, they get stumped. "I don't think I'm a genius at anything," they tell me.

Well, then let's start with an easier question. What are you good at that makes you happy? When I was working at Ford Motor Company, I had a friend who was really good at working on alternators and motors and all of that. He always said how dumb he was, but I had a different point of view. I told him,

"When you open the hood of a car, you see the engine and all the intricate pieces of that motor and car that I could never see." We had this conversation several times, and eventually he started to see himself as a genius in that realm. That's the discovery you are looking for. Sometimes you need someone else to notice it first.

When you look at the origin of the word *genius*, you'll see that at first it wasn't associated with an *unusual* ability. It just referred to an innate ability. Here's one of the definitions of genius from Merriam-Webster: "a peculiar, distinctive, or identifying character or spirit."[2] We all have an identifying character or spirit. Maybe yours is finding beauty in nature. Maybe it's compassion for the underdog. Maybe you have an uncanny ability to be curious. Maybe you remember songs after hearing them only one time. We all have a genius based in the original meaning of the word—a distinctive trait. But we all have genius in the current understanding of the word as well—something to offer the world that no one else can offer.

When I think of my distinctive trait and what I offer that no one else can, I see that my genius is relationship building and engagement. I grew up in the farming community of Arkansas City, Kansas. It was predominantly white, but I had a small, tight-knit community of African American uncles and aunts. We weren't necessarily related, but from a young age everyone around me embodied a collectiveness without articulating it.

Since I was little I had worked on Uncle Will's farm. He

didn't hesitate to give me a kick in the pants. "Biggun, you're gonna have to work harder than that," he'd say if he caught me slowing down. Uncle Will was there for the fun times too. No one needed an invite to our family BBQ. If my grandfather was out in the BBQ pit, you showed up for ribs, burgers, hot dogs, and Bev's famous potato salad.

Uncle Will's kids—my cousins—were always there. I didn't find out until later I wasn't related to them by blood, that Uncle Will wasn't my father's actual brother. There was never a distinction between my cousins by blood—who were there too—and the cousins related by something just as strong. There were so many forces against us, we all had to stick together. I learned how to relate with family members of all ages, how to connect within a community. Because of this foundation I've always had a sense of being part of something bigger.

I wasn't always clear on my genius, but I am now. Knowing my genius allows me to use it to benefit others, and I find that work deeply satisfying. I hope I can be a positive influence on my patients and players and, in the personal realm, on my friends and relatives. I think that's the best hope any of us have of making an impact on the world—by influencing our immediate networks.

Before you can share your genius with your network and the world, you need to find out what it is. To identify your genius, first think about yourself. What do you like to do? What comes naturally? When do the hours slip by? Hungarian

American psychologist Mihaly Csikszentmihalyi talked about flow, that hyper-mental focus and immersion. When do you feel totally immersed in and absorbed by what you're doing? When do things flow?

Sometimes a skill comes easily, but it's not your passion. If it's not your passion, it's probably not the kind of genius I'm talking about here. Choose a particular skill or impulse where you have a lot to contribute and where you also enjoy making that contribution. Once you alight on your genius, you can start devoting yourself to it and, hopefully, using it to help others.

You may well have a genius that doesn't present itself in a class-room. Think about the roles that come naturally to you when you're in a group. Are you the person who comes up with an idea for the weekend? Do you make plans happen by handling logistics and keeping things organized? Are you a peacemaker? Are you the person who keeps up the momentum of the conversation? Do you love the spotlight? Do you have a talent for helping other people shine?

Think of someone you know with a clear genius. What is their genius? Do you know when they discovered it? (If you can ask, go ahead and do so.) Do they use it to help others? How?

For the next few days, start keeping track of moments where you seem to handle things effortlessly. Does anything jump out at you as an area you'd like to explore further?

Sometimes we need someone's help to discover our genius. Ask a trusted friend or mentor what they perceive your strengths to be. They don't have to be someone with a deep personal knowl-edge of your life. Sometimes a new perspective can be helpful too. You might be surprised at the answers.

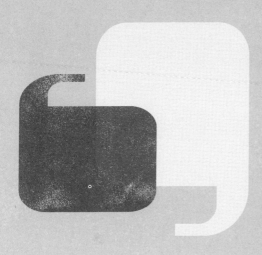

I think that's the best hope any of us have of making an impact on the world—by influencing our immediate networks.

How much time do you spend looking in the mirror?

For most people, I think the answer here is going to be, "Very little or none." I hope to change that. Looking in the mirror is an opportunity to see yourself as a separate person, to be curious, to learn.

The mirror is where I bring many of my practices. Visualization. Personification. Diving deep into the root of current patterns. Increasing awareness. It might feel weird at first to face yourself in this way, but it's a process, and like any practice, it gets easier the more you do it.

A few days ago I had an intense travel schedule coming up for work, but my youngest son, Azrie, had a football game midweek. Fitting in the game would have meant two early morning flights and a bit of juggling to catch back up with the Pistons. My first thought was I had to miss the game. But then I looked in the mirror. The guy in the mirror had a broader perspective. He wasn't worried about losing a little sleep and dealing with some sprints from one gate to another. He was thinking bigger. *What will your sons say when you're no longer here? What will they recall about Dad? Will they say, "He was really busy, but he always made a way to be supportive and be around"?*

I could have avoided the mirror. I could have told my son I wasn't going to make it. My son would have been okay. But the guy in the mirror would have been disappointed. That voice was clear. *Do you know how important it will be for Azrie to know you left the road trip and came home to see him play?* That was the mirror working and pushing me.

When you're engaged with the mirror, you can test out your value system, and try on different choices and imagine how they play out. What does a choice say about who you are and what you value? The mirror is a safe place to improvise. It's a chance to have a conversation with yourself about who you want to be and to try inhabiting that new role.

If you recoil at the idea of facing yourself, think about why that might be. Why do you avoid the mirror? Many times, when you get in front of the mirror, you're going to be challenged with who you are and who you want to be. Sometimes there's a world of difference between those, and this can be uncomfortable. You might not like what the person in the mirror tells you. But I believe in the verse from the book of John that says, "The truth will set you free." You have to get to the truth first before you can make a change. Try it—lean in, be curious, ask one question after another.

Embrace the tension, because this is where you're going to change. As you continually show up to do this reflective work, your inner self will become more congruent with that person in the mirror. You'll start to feel the two entities almost blend into one being. The mirror is the gateway to inner harmony.

So take the opportunity today to look at you—*your truest you*—and just be curious. And hey, you may find out you're pretty great company.

TELL YOUR STORY

Step in front of a mirror, and look at that person. Try to notice the first word that comes to your mind. The words will come quickly, so pay attention. Hold onto that very first word, and become curious about it. What are the textures of that word? What emotions does it evoke? How does your body feel when you say it aloud? Repeat this practice every day, and track your thoughts in a journal. At the end of a week, look for common textures and tones of the words that arise.

Take a look at yourself in the mirror. Notice your expression. Now smile. Is it a genuine smile? If not, what would it take to make it genuine? What do you like about the person you see? Keep coming back, starting with a smile, and seek out one kind observation each and every day. I promise, it gets easier.

As you look at yourself in the mirror, try to envision your reflection as a separate person. Do you feel compassion toward that person, or do you notice criticisms racing to the surface? Can you embrace that person staring back at you? Do you believe he or she has the answers you need?

Where are your sacred spaces?

Y ou know I love the mirror. To me, it is a sacred space. There's no one else around, just me and the man who stares back at me. Another sacred space is my chocolate-brown leather chair. It sits in the living room, kind of central in the home, with a huge storage ottoman, where I keep all my notes and a pen. From the chair I have a view of the maple trees outside. I watch the green buds on the trees in the spring and the crispy, orange leaves falling in October.

"That's dad's space," the kids say. They know. The chair is connected to deep, comforting feelings of having my family around. We have had many hard and great conversations around that chair. This is a place I love myself and protect what gives me comfort, so it's also a place where I draw a line. The kids sometimes want to sit there, but it's a good lesson for them that they can't. They know this place is my sanctuary, where I can come recharge and reconnect with my values. They know my self-care goes hand in hand with nurturing them, so they have grown to respect that I'm going to protect this space for myself. A healthier me will make for a healthier family in the long run.

Hanging on a wall near the chair is a picture of wolves traveling in the snow, probably thirty of them in a line. I found it at the Minnesota State Fair. It makes me think of my family—my kinship family—traveling together in an often-hostile environment. I know if something threatens our pack, I can step in. That role as protector is sacred to me.

I've got other sacred spaces.

The football field. That was a place where I could be aggressive and get rewarded for it. I could get out all of the stuff that was bottled up over years and take it out in the game. I had been told by my mother and grandmother that as a big, dark-skinned man I would be seen as a threat. I had to be gentle and articulate. I could never raise my voice. That was them protecting me. But the football field was one place I didn't need protection.

A sacred place doesn't have to be static or singular. For some people it's sitting on a train watching the landscape go by. For others it's being at a concert, listening to live guitar. You might associate a sacred space with a spiritual place or a location in nature. It might be where you can be at peace and connected to the world outside yourself. Certain majestic spaces are almost sacred by nature. The ocean. The mountains. The forest. These may remind you that the world is bigger than your daily worries, and give you hope that it's possible to change the path you're on. But you don't need something as grand as the redwoods to make you feel connected to life in a more meaningful way. Maybe there's a fountain in your neighborhood that reminds you that the world is fluid, always in motion, full of hope. Maybe you have a special tree in your yard, providing shelter and a sense of rootedness.

Lock into the spaces where concerns fly away and where peace reigns. And when you find one, name it and protect it. When a sacred place chooses you, it's your task to keep it sacred.

TELL YOUR STORY

Draw a sketch of your sacred space. Don't worry about the quality of the drawing. What are some of the features of your sacred space? What does it allow you to see? What are the emotions you associate with that space? Can you go there physically, or is it some place you imagine?

Are there any photographs, objects, or pieces of art that mean a great deal to you? Something that illuminates a deeper truth about your life? This thing may be stunning, it may be odd, it may be objectively ugly. But something that reminds you of who you are is infinitely more valuable than a pretty object in the house.

As you make some of the centering practices part of your daily routine, you may start to associate a certain space with the clarity and sense of connectedness you gain by tuning in there. Maybe pick a spot in the house where you can regularly pause, take some centering breaths, reflect, and allow yourself to dive deep. This is a kind of devotion. A sense of sacredness will begin to accrue.

Do you know how to do battle?

Y ou may have heard of the term *cognitive dissonance*. In music, dissonance involves clashing notes, something discordant. It's unpleasant, the opposite of harmonious. Based on this definition you may think of cognitive dissonance as negative. But I want to give you a new way to think about it.

One dissonant memory that stands out in my life happened early on in my marriage with Carrie. She was pregnant with our first son, Izaiah, and one evening at dinner, her mother prompted us with a question about how we would discipline him. Now what you have to understand is that I came from an authoritarian family. I grew up in a family that spanked, and it worked out pretty well for me. You did what you're told, no room for asking too many questions. Carrie experienced the opposite in her childhood—more of a democratic approach to parenting.

This question from Carrie's mom brought a battle to the surface. This happened early in our relationship—just about six months after our wedding—and I still wanted to impress Carrie's family. So for the duration of the dinner, I kept my contentiousness below the surface. But we all knew it was brewing. We left dinner, and Carrie and I knew we needed to battle it out to figure out which approach we were going to follow.

Over the next few months, I explained my views about the value of firm parenting. I had strong opinions about how to raise Black children and believed a disciplinarian hand was necessary at times. That's a unique and valuable perspective I brought to the conversation. Carrie also reflected on what mattered most in her democratic family environment. In the battle we were both able to better articulate our *why*. It caused us to bring our subconscious values up to the surface. And because of the battle, we were then able to come together early in our marriage to create a new agenda, informed by our pasts, but something altogether new. The battle brought about a new version of *us*.

Some of us run at the first sign of tension. The problem feels too hard to solve. The options are too dissonant. But I'm here to tell you that you have to stay and fight. Battling helps us bring "deep down" up to the surface, helping you become more aware of what's really shaping your decisions.

The battle is what you want. That may feel counterintuitive, but battling out your value statements yields clarity. If you keep things below the level of conscious awareness, you won't see the conflict. It will stay hidden. But doing battle with yourself and others helps you become aware of your values. The battle gives you more control of the life you are choosing.

The battle gives you a chance to tell a different story than the one you are used to telling. When you're battling with yourself or someone else, you're regaining awareness of what's driving you underneath. You're finding your power. You're finding your new way of living. It's not easy. (Growth almost never is.) Let the battle reveal who you are, clarify how your choices and values align, and sharpen your vision of who you want to be.

TELL YOUR STORY

What battle needs to take place today? Think of an area of your life where you're experiencing tension with another person in your personal life. Grab a journal, and list all the reasons that you feel strongly about your approach. Just keep asking *why*. That one little word is your shovel, digging up layer by layer of your past. Think back on your childhood, your values, your experiences, your views on race, politics, religion—whatever it is that's really driving you.

Now turn the page and write down the opposing point of view, and try to get in the head of whomever you're doing battle with. Consider what may be motivating their opinion. Have you ever asked them? If not, try to find time this week to better understand their *why*.

Once you have both of your *whys* on the page, now is the time to accommodate, listen, and compromise. It may take a few small battles before we finish the war, and that's okay. That's what you want. Keep coming back—not to wear down one another—but rather, to stir up all the stories that are underneath. Share your awareness with one another. Battle it out.

What are the challenges you face in your life?

Fifteen years ago, when my youngest son was one year old, I realized I had a problem. Actually, I had a bunch of problems, but at the center was one big one that made all the others much harder—I drank too much. I wasn't awake to my life.

Drinking was a linchpin problem. Everything else was affected by it. When I stopped drinking, I stopped smoking and a multiplicity of other struggles started to subside. My health improved. My kidney function was better. My blood pressure went down too. I saved a ton of money by not going out and drinking with friends. Most importantly, I became more available for my family.

Instead of spending Saturday nights out with friends, I was

hanging out with Carrie and the boys. Plus, I was no longer hungover on Sundays. That meant I could go to the swimming pool in the summer with the boys, which they loved. I splashed around in the water with abandon while metaphorically I was finally back on dry land. I didn't realize I'd been holding my breath all those years. I'd been underwater. When I stopped drinking, I could breathe. All these positive changes stemmed from addressing the linchpin issue of drinking.

I'm a therapist so I'm used to hearing about challenges. They come in all shapes and sizes. But I can give you advice that will apply to most all of the challenges you face. First, look for the linchpin problem and focus your energy there. Second, take small steps.

Big problem, small steps.

My first small step to address my drinking problem was inviting my wife into the process. She was the only one who knew I'd made the decision to quit. She became my support system, as I increasingly rejected calls from friends who centered their lives on alcohol. She listened as I explained how awkward I felt socializing with my peers, always defending why I didn't want to have a sip. Having her as my "sponsor" made these small steps more doable.

We all are going to face challenges—some big and some small. Instead of taking the path of least resistance or avoiding the discomfort of telling the truth about ourselves and others, we can face those challenges head on. We can invite others into the process, to feel a little less alone. The discomfort of vulnerability is how we move forward, develop, and make changes, little by little. There is no magic pill for any of these changes.

There's an African saying—*How do you eat an elephant?* The answer is one bite at a time. Big problem, little bites, people.

TELL YOUR STORY

What are you challenged with today? Make a list. Write down three to five challenges you currently face. Now look at the list. Are any items connected? Are some bigger than others? Look at the intersection of how your challenges relate to one another.

Circle one of the problems that might be a linchpin, and start there. Let's try to get to the root. When looking at your linchpin problem, ask yourself when it began. Were there people who helped it grow or fester? Write the story around the first time you experienced this problem.

Think back to your genius and the things about yourself that make you proud. What specific strengths can you draw on to help you meet a challenge?

Now let's try a bite-sized approach to addressing this challenge. What's one small step you can take today? What's even *the* smallest step? If you want to manage your time better, maybe it's buying a planner. If you want to improve a relationship, maybe it's picking up the phone. If it's a diet, maybe it's finding one recipe and making a list of ingredients.

With feedback from those who you trust the most, and time for reflection to hear your own thoughts, you can make progress today on one of the biggest challenges you face. That would be quite an accomplishment for the day, in my book.

How can your vulnerability free you?

When I began my PhD journey, I wasn't a great writer. Suddenly I found myself at an R1 institute,[3] churning out research-based writing. In general, I would grasp the concepts fairly easily, but communicating my ideas in a technical way was a hell of a struggle. My first thought was to hide that. I couldn't let on that the writing piece was killing me. I was the first person in my family to go to college, and here I was a doctoral candidate. I had to just keep moving along. Researching concepts, taking notes, positing theories, synthesizing ideas, and churning out papers. So I kept my head down in the books and kept banging away at the keyboard. If I could keep my weaknesses from my advisor, Dr. Doherty—if I could keep the conversation lively enough and full of my usual self-deprecating jokes—maybe he wouldn't notice.

But my wife kept it real. "You're not going to be able to hide the inability to write in a PhD program," she told me. "Not happening. Everybody's going to know." I knew she was right. I sought out my advisor and I confessed I really struggled with writing.

"I know," he said, not missing a beat. "I'm reading your stuff." So that was a bit comical. And embarrassing. But you know what it was more than anything? It was freeing. I was truth telling. And I was setting myself free.

Sure, it took some energy to face up to the truth at first. But it paid me back with interest. I was doing ten times the work to try to cover the "secret" about my writing. When I let myself be vulnerable, named the problem, and shared the struggle, I transferred it outside of me. There was an emotional release even that first moment just in naming the struggle.

Under Dr. Doherty's tutelage (and with the help of my wife), I got better at writing the way we get better at almost everything—by doing a hell of a lot of it and taking in continuous feedback. "Write like crazy," Dr. Doherty told me. "Then give it to me. I'm going to mark it up and you're going to write it again." He wouldn't just mark up my paper. He would tear it up, red pen marks everywhere. But I never felt bad about that because I knew he was helping me, just like the coaches had helped me get better when I played football. In both cases, I trusted these people because I'd come to know and respect them. That created space for me to be comfortable and vulnerable.

Many of us resist vulnerability. But if you want to change or grow, you have to first become aware of those inner places of insecurity, weakness, and embarrassment. Then you have to put them all out in front of yourself and name them. They don't define you. This is just one aspect of your character, that's all. You have many others, and a lot of our work in this book is to identify and celebrate your many strengths. That helps to counterbalance the acknowledgement of your weaknesses.

In her book *The Power of Vulnerability*, Brené Brown talks about vulnerability and its intersection with courage. You have to draw on your inner strength and say, *Okay, I'm ready to be a beginner.* You have to have the courage to admit there is an area where you're not as strong, which, paradoxically, takes strength. Open yourself up to vulnerability; so much power awaits on the other side.

TELL YOUR STORY

What's something you want to get better at? Or what are some qualities or skills you're embarrassed you don't yet possess?

Grab your journal and write whatever comes to mind. How long have you been avoiding this task? Is it a long time? Why have you been avoiding it? Is there a deeper fear under the surface? If so, write down your fears.

That fear is now outside of you. And now that it's in the open, we can start to tackle it.

As we've seen, vulnerability and growth is a group project. Here are tips for identifying individuals who can walk with you through your vulnerability:

- They're freewheeling with kindness. You've noticed their propensity for calling out goodness in others.
- They have skills and qualities you desire to develop.
- They have a sense of humor.
- They have margin in their schedule to mentor you well.

Think about the people in your life, including the ones you don't necessarily consider close friends. Are there any good candidates for accompanying you on this walk?

Conversely, identify areas where you feel confident, where you know what you're doing. Be on the lookout. You never know when someone may be looking to you to usher them through their own vulnerabilities with kind words and candor.

What untruths are you telling yourself about your current existence?

I n my midthirties I was married with two boys and working at Ford Motor Company. I was happy with my job. It was physical work, and my existence on the planet up to that point had all been rooted in my physical strength (remember how I got started on football?).

My wife had other ideas. She started pushing me toward education, which was a foreign language to me. I hadn't even graduated from Long Beach State because I was going to be a pro football player. "Not a chance I'm going back to school," I told my wife. For years I had been telling myself that my existence was physical, not intellectual. But at Ford I became a union rep and started working on its diversity program. It got me thinking, *Maybe there is another path for me.*

What untruths are you telling yourself about your daily existence? Or, like me at age thirty-five, about your entire life thus far?

My wife wouldn't let up with her daily drumbeat about school. She saw a talent within me I couldn't visualize, and she didn't want me to live an unexplored life in the fog. She intuitively knew graduate school was the next frontier for me, to explore another genius she knew I possessed. I wasn't so sure, so I told her if she gathered all my transcripts and paperwork, I'd do it.

Man, is she persistent.

I found myself taking night classes at Metropolitan State University after a ten-hour shift at Ford, and later I studied at the University of Minnesota. I fell in love with psychology—in particular, community psychology. I was worried I might quickly fall behind. Instead, when we started studying systems thinking, the concept came naturally to me. This was how I had always seen the world. I observed people and looked for patterns and interactions, and the forces and structures that guided those patterns and interactions. In my coursework I was given the terminology for what I'd always understood.

It turns out, I *absolutely* belonged at this institution. Being defined solely by my physical stature was a deeply rooted untruth. The other students weren't any smarter than me.

They'd just spent more time in their minds. Turns out, I could do that too.

Jean-Paul Sartre was a French existentialist philosopher who was intrigued by ideas of freedom and choice. "Man is condemned to be free," he said in a 1945 lecture given in Paris. At first that statement might sound puzzling. Being condemned is a bad thing, but freedom is good, right? What Sartre understood is that we tell ourselves untruths to avoid facing the alternatives. True freedom—the ability to make your own choices—is a heavy responsibility. "I have to stay in a relationship because of the kids" or "I have to stay in this job to pay the bills." There may be other options, but we don't want to consider them. It's more comfortable to pretend we don't have other options.

The truth is, you can make changes, but you're going to have to deal with the consequences of those changes. Saying you have only one option is a cop-out—just a way to make yourself believe you don't have a choice. In fact, you do.

Ford ended up closing its plant and gave offers to employees to fund a return to school or get a payout of $100,000. I took the scholarship and went for my master's. I became a Presidential Leadership Scholar. I got straight As. I was the first in my family to get a bachelor's degree, and then I went past my master's to get a PhD in one of the top programs in the world.

When I rejected the lie that I was just a strong, physical guy and embraced my potential, I opened up an entirely new path.

I had to face up to my fears and insecurities. In some ways it would have been easier to stay with my original story. I could have stayed in my comfort zone. But when I started exploring my PhD, professors saw that I was serious, that I was ready to make the effort. They saw me show up and make changes for myself, and that made them want to help me.

Some of you may discover your untruths early in life, but for many people, like me, that plot twist happens a little later. The great news is that it's never too late. When you uncover your untruths, you can begin to flourish. Not *instantly*, but that stark moment of discovery is the beginning of a rewarding journey. When it arrives, don't turn your back on it.

TELL YOUR STORY

Where are you not telling the truth to yourself? Where are you holding yourself back from a growth opportunity?

As you ask these questions, notice if you start to feel tense or uncomfortable. Notice if you have an urge to jump out of your seat. This could be a good indicator that you're on the verge of uncovering a lie you tell yourself. It's in this sticky, vulnerable place that you're going to grow. Do yourself a favor—stay there, in that moment, and talk it out with yourself.

You don't need to quit your job today or put your house on the market. All we're doing is starting to speak the truth aloud. Telling yourself the truth about who you are and what you want is the cornerstone to all your work.

Where are you acting in bad faith in terms of the available options? Sometimes untruths arise because we're not taking the time to be creative. Sometimes we tell ourselves there are no other paths or choices because we're repeating the behaviors modeled by those around us. So let's get creative! Get in the playground!

Think about one area of your life where you feel you're at the end of a road. As fast as you can, write down ten choices you could make that would get you unstuck. A choice that would help transform a negative space into a positive one. A choice that would allow you to escape a place that's bad for you. A choice that would bring power back into your locus of control. Even if these hypothetical choices feel irrational or impossible, just for this exercise, I want you to entertain what *could* happen.

Look at your list. Sure, none of those ten choices may be good or wise right now, but be encouraged—you have the power to make choices. Here in the playground, you just found ten examples of power available to you. This kind of creativity will carry you far.

What is your essence?

The words that describe us change over time, but certain overarching words or descriptions may ring true forever. Beginning in my teenage years, before I had any idea what therapy was, I began to play the role of connector with friends and family. I was a good listener. I was gentle. I brought people together. But I wasn't afraid of conflict either. I was a good go-between. I believe that word *connector* is the overarching essence of who I am. Every "genius" I've ever had falls under this descriptor.

Fast-forward to college football. NFL scouts would give us feedback as to how they saw us fitting into the NFL. The coaches would then take that feedback and use it to guide us. Some players struggled with that process, and it would sometimes create friction between players and coaches. I was always comfortable mediating in these circumstances. I would help players understand what they were being asked to do. Coaches began to notice that ability and would come to me asking for help. "Jason is not getting this," they'd say. "Can you talk to him? Help him better understand why we're asking what we're asking." I was happy to be the conduit. It was part of my essence.

Another area that's always been comfortable involves big ideas. I love them. I'm good at the big picture, thinking of possibilities. But there's a flip side of that quality—I am not detail oriented. People say that about me all the time, and I can't fight them on that. I'm great at the big picture. Details, not so much. So how do I play to my strengths and minimize my weaknesses? Discovering the essence of who you are also means discovering who you aren't. On a basketball court the paint shows us what is in bounds and what is out. The same concept is at work here. We see what we are because of the contrast to what we are not.

In my doctoral pursuit I had to refocus and reframe. I had no choice but to start paying better attention to details. But I also had to strategize by finding someone to whom details came naturally and do two things: (1) learn from that person and (2) leverage our relationship so our natural strengths could complement each other. It was sometimes just a matter of asking directly. *Can you help me with this detailed space? And when you want help brainstorming, connecting, spinning out possibilities, I'm your guy.*

I'm very fortunate that I have this dynamic with my

wife—where I'm weak, she's strong. Where she's weak, I'm strong. The essence of who I am is balanced by my wife's essence. That's helped us become more tightly woven; we're better off together. (It also helps to remember that during some of our tenser conversations.) I didn't have to reinvent myself as this brand-new, detail-oriented person, and she knows that the devil can be in the details. She knows how to stay there and make ideas operational.

Your essence will be an enduring quality in your life, regardless of circumstances, and once you start to identify it, it can make you feel centered. It will be a tether when you step into new places and new challenges. Often, when our essence is on display, we feel most authentic, and others sense that too.

TELL YOUR STORY

In your journal chart three moments in your life. Now observe those stories as if you were a first-time viewer. Is there an underlying theme? This may help you reveal your essence.

Try a cluster technique to generate words to describe yourself. Start in the middle of the page with one word that describes you in some fundamental way. Draw a circle around the word, draw a line out, then draw another circle. Put a word in the next circle that the first word made you think of. Keep freely associating words and connecting them to each other with lines and circles until you draw a blank. Then go back to the word in the center and start another branch of circles.

Don't worry if a word pops into your mind that doesn't seem to fit or doesn't seem related. Let your mind wander and make its own associations. Write down whatever comes. When our minds spark in different directions, we don't always know what's behind it. Trust your intuition. It could be leading somewhere interesting.

When you finish, review the words. Which of these descriptors buoy you? Which ones bring you down?

It's also helpful to hear how others describe us. Ask those close to you what words they'd use to describe you. Do you laugh in recognition? Bristle at characterizations that aren't particularly appealing? If you hear words that don't feel right, this gives you the opportunity to push in the other direction.

If some traits that feel negative pop up in how you or others describe you, don't stuff them away just yet. Can you take those and turn them around, finding the positive trait contained within it? For example, if people say you're impulsive, are you also spontaneous—someone who steals the show when it's time to brainstorm? If you're anxious, are you conscientious and concerned about others? If you're rigid, are you good at protecting your time? Spinning the word around doesn't mean you don't want to change, but it means you can come at the trait from another angle and perhaps bring out the positive side.

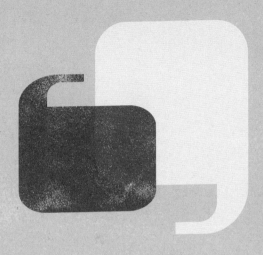

Trust your intuition. It could be leading somewhere interesting.

Can you let go of negative patterns you developed in childhood?

A coach once told me he remembered his anxiety starting when he was nine or ten. He had a natural talent for basketball, and after a few impressive games, expectations skyrocketed. Being really good wasn't enough. He had to be the *best*. Anxiety pushed him to be the best player on the court. Now he's a coach, and his career on the court is done. Does he need to hold on to that anxiety from childhood? Or can he let it go?

In my practice I often notice roots of anxiety and depression originating in those tumultuous teen years. It's also when many individuals begin developing passive-aggressive behavior because they realize aggressive behavior won't be tolerated by the adults in their lives. Even being direct is often met with discomfort, so many people start developing a lack of clarity, especially in stating or even being aware of their own needs.

Whatever the case may be, the pain of challenging experiences in our childhood and teen years often leads to patterns in our adult lives that no longer serve us. Once upon a time, they protected us. Now, as we faithfully do our self-inventory work, we realize we can let some of those behaviors go.

How do we do that? Let's take anxiety as an example, as it's a common struggle and one we can at least partially address in a small space. I like to describe anxiety as an unwanted friend. We've all had friends visit who outstayed their welcome. The meal is over. Dessert is done. The sink is piled high with dishes, and the candles are starting to burn out. But that friend is simply hunkered deep into your couch yapping away with one or two stories on heavy rotation. She has absolutely no sense that you're ready to call it a night.

Anxiety can be useful. For example, it can push us to study for an exam. And this friend has good qualities too—that's why you are friends. She's always up for getting together, and can be a great storyteller when she's not repeating herself. But this show's over. So what will you do? You tell her. "Tomorrow's a big day. I gotta shut this down."

By personifying anxiety, you bring it under your control. It is not some nebulous outside force, like an unexpected rain shower that ruins a picnic. It's merely a friend who had a little too much sauvignon blanc and isn't reading the room correctly. Open the door, send her on her way, and hand her an umbrella if necessary.

If you can personify an issue, it's taken outside you. It doesn't define you; it's just someone who comes to visit. Remember when I said at the start of the book that we were going to go down to the roots and start yanking? Well it's time to get out the gardening gloves (and maybe some kneepads).

TELL YOUR STORY

Let's use the playground to go back in time and get inside the sixteen-year-old version of you. Draw or write as much as you can remember about the following questions:

What house did you live in?
What was your bedroom like?
Can you imagine yourself walking inside?
Is anyone in there, or are you alone?
What color are the walls?
What does it sound like? Is there music? A TV? Loud neighbors?
Imagine taking a seat on your bed. What's the predominant emotional experience that comes to mind? Anxiety, depression, aggression, or something else?

Now try personifying that emotion. Imagine the textures, colors, and smells. Maybe even draw a picture of it. If you like, take a moment to write a letter to the person you were when this emotion began. Writing letters gives you a chance to honor who you were and how you have grown and developed beyond that person who stood on the precipice of the adult world.

Now that you've taken time to honor your former self, turn your attention back to the present. Do you need this emotion anymore? Or do you have new tools to protect and preserve yourself?

Let's try the personification exercise I described above with anxiety as a friend and apply it to a pattern you would like to change. Can you think of a character that represents the feeling or behavior? Thank him for his time and tell him to go sit down now.

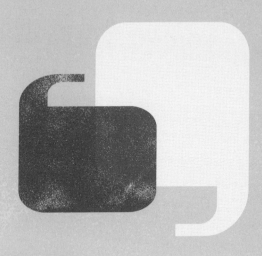

By personifying anxiety, you
bring it under your control.

What makes you deeply happy?

When I was in my twenties, drinking Coors Light with my buddies and paying for everyone's drinks made me happy. That wouldn't make me happy today at all. In fact, I usually avoid that space of drinking with friends. Today spending time with my wife and my boys makes me happy. There's nothing I like more than hanging out by the grill together with the smoker going, the folks my sons call their uncles coming by for ribs and chicken, a Chiefs game on in the background.

My work makes me happy too. Reading about racial and ethnic relationships, discovering research on socialization patterns or self-talk that may help me offer better support to others—I find a great deal of satisfaction in that. And you may have guessed by now that I'm hooked on stimulating conversation. I get a spark from those *aha* moments in conversation and therapy. But even ten years ago, none of those things would have been on my list (except conversations—I always loved those).

Happiness is something that we all seek—weekly, daily, moment to moment. What makes you feel happy? It's a question that seems simple. But when you scratch beneath the surface, it can almost stump you. People turn to ancient philosophy to make them happy. Positive psychology. The Danish lifestyle.

Happiness is a relative term, and your relationship to this word will shift over time. My players have achieved much of what society tells us will make us happy. Success, fame, fortune, the house of their dreams. But some of them tell me the mansion didn't bring happiness. Being a celebrity didn't bring happiness. Neither did the pool with the waterfall or even the views of the ocean. Somewhere in the back of their minds they knew the promises of wealth and fame bringing happiness weren't true.

So what is it? *What is happiness?*

You know, I don't know.

Defining happiness can be slippery, so rather than forcing a concrete definition, I find this concept is best revealed in *contrast.* You can recognize a state of feeling happy by comparing it to times when you are sad or disappointed.

In my life I understand deep happiness as it relates to pain.

I lost my dad at the age of fifteen. After that, at our football games, I'd hear my friends' fathers telling them, "Son, you got this." The words almost physically hurt, but I learned how to slip away, or perhaps that's when I began slipping underwater. But because of that loss, I can connect with young men who didn't have fathers in their lives. I'm happy that I can produce spaces for younger Black boys to share their struggles. I'm present with them in their suffering, and that is gratifying to me. But the root of that present fulfillment stems from the internal chaos of my fifteen-year-old self. Would I feel this unbridled happiness if I hadn't had the contrast of unbridled sadness? If it hadn't grown directly *from* that sadness?

So instead of looking to transitory things that supposedly make you happy, I'd encourage you to look at those spaces that hold pain, sadness, or loss, and see if you, too, can find happiness that may bud from that root.

What you need even more than happiness is fulfillment—something that goes deep into who you are and why you're on this earth.

Consider where you have felt pain and suffering. Are there branches of happiness that grew out of those painful roots? How have you been able to connect with others over a shared pain point? How has suffering helped you develop a deeper trust in yourself? Has your pain revealed a passion or calling that allows you to give back to others?

Make a list of things that make you deeply happy. This is not simply a space of feeling entertained or an escape from anxiety, but things that connect to the core of who you are and how you want to spend your life. When you have a list of what makes you deeply happy, make a goal to maximize your presence with the people, relationships, and causes that help you experience that fulfillment.

Take a look at your calendar. Seek out those fulfilling things! If your current calendar is devoid of the opportunities you just defined, then maybe it's worth asking yourself if significant career or relational changes are on the horizon.

Do you ruminate on things in your past or in your future?

Just mentioning the words *depression* and *anxiety* might make your tense shoulders clench up to your ears, but I'd like to approach this conversation with a little less pressure. Instead of labeling yourself with depression or anxiety—as so many of us do—for the purpose of this book we're going to simply become aware of our subconscious thoughts. Specifically, our unconscious propensity to drift away from the present.

In layman's terms, depression is ruminating on something that has happened in the past. Anxiety is worrying about something that may happen in the future. Now obviously the therapeutic definitions are much more complex, but the past-future explanations give us a simple entryway into complicated topics.

In contrast to visualization, which is the intentional reflection we've already discussed, anxiety and depression are marked by out-of-control ruminations and fixations. In visualization, you're in control and it's productive. Rumination is unproductive, and it leaves you feeling out of control. It's a broken record. It's a basketball player thinking to himself, *Coach is gonna take me out. My contract is coming up. I'm going to screw this up,* over and over with no progress and no attempt at problem-solving. It's being stuck in a loop of unproductive thoughts.

You may feel anxiety in your body before you can even name it. Increased heart rate, clammy hands, a change in energy. Tune in to these physical changes, and notice the thoughts that are paired with them. You may be surprised at the inner monologue occurring. Many of us invent stories based in fear about what horrible things *could* happen, but the lie of anxiety is that this imagined future *is guaranteed* to happen. Challenge that monologue with questions rooted in your present reality.

If you've dealt with anxiety your entire life, you're not going to suddenly catch it and stop it every time, but by practicing these things you will start to become more aware. Similarly with depression, you're not going to catch yourself slumped over on the bed, exhausted, and recognize depression and immediately pull yourself out of it. But you can start to ask the right questions.

When you feel yourself ruminating about either the past or the future, I want you create a mantra, which is a self-soothing technique. A mantra is a form of self-talk that you take into battle to remind you of who you are. It's like a long rope tethering you to the present when you are being knocked around in the waves of anxiety and depression.

I don't want to tell you what your mantra should be, but I'll give you an example. Let's take a basketball player who is not shooting the percentage he wants to from the free throw line. He wants to get better. There are all kinds of technical things he can use to get better. But a mantra can help too. It complements that technical and physical work.

"I was built for this. I'm gonna make this."

Or maybe you struggle with weight loss and find yourself unable to think positively when you start exercising. How about one of these mantras? "That's okay. I'm going to be all right. Change doesn't happen overnight." Or "That's okay. I don't have to lose it all today."

It's gentleness on repeat, designed to bring you back to now. Your power in these moments will be found in excavating kind truths about yourself. A mantra helps you stay in the moment. The only true thing we have in our life is this moment. What we talked about twelve minutes ago is gone forever. What we will talk about in ten minutes is yet to be determined. Don't let today be consumed by every other day. And remember, in staying present and gentle, there is power.

TELL YOUR STORY

Think of five possible mantras for yourself. Keep them short—about seven words is a good length. Say each one aloud. Which one feels the best for this moment? Make any adjustments you want to make, and start saying it over and over.

As you practice the mantra, gently ask yourself: *How is my breathing? Am I staying in this current moment?*

Now that you've practiced the mantra sitting still, try it while you're doing something where you need the affirmation. Maybe it's on the way to the doctor's office. Or to a meeting. Or to a family dinner with a relative whose politics differ from yours. Use your mantra to remind yourself to breathe, stay gentle, and remember how powerful you are.

What are you proudest of about yourself?

L et's keep feeling good about ourselves. We're on a roll. How do you react when I say the word *pride*?

Pride is something many of us find tricky. We don't want to be too prideful in ourselves. After all, arrogance is never appealing. I'm talking not about hubris. I'm talking about pride that's earned the old-fashioned way, by working to reach your potential. It's easy for me to be proud of what my sons have accomplished, or my players or patients. I celebrate them every day. I have no trouble there, but it's harder to recognize my own accomplishments, although I'm getting better at it.

I'm proud of how I've modeled hard work for my sons. Growing up, all they knew was Dad sitting in the den with two laptops, an array of highlighters, books, and articles, continuously pursuing new knowledge. I believe my wife and I, both working and pursuing degrees, have given our boys a strong work ethic. I'm also both proud and nervous that they've developed a high level of Black consciousness. The world will see that as a threat. (Pride is not always simple. Few things are for a Black man in America.)

When it comes to the professional arena, I'm proud that my accomplishments better position me to help others. A lot of my happiness is rooted in seeing others' joy around me, and my pride is rooted in the same space. My task in this life on earth is to be supportive of others. I'm proud that I can create a safe space relatively quickly. I'm proud that people feel they can talk to me about things. That they don't feel judged. I'm proud that the players on the Pistons feel comfortable around me. That they see me as a role model who is always available for them, always approachable.

We all have natural strengths and abilities. We explored some of this in the question about your genius. But your pride really stems from the places *where you put in the work*. In this section I want you to go a little further, reflecting back on your hard work and not just celebrating natural abilities. A professor told me a long time ago, "Be careful saying you're a natural anything, because if it seems natural it means you put in a hell of a lot of work for it to seem that way." Be proud of the work, the successes, and the stumbles as well.

I talk about this with my players. When you have an elite

shooter, people call him a natural. The way the ball leaves his hands, the way it sails through the air. Yes indeed, he's a force of nature. A born talent. He has a genius.

But here's where pride comes into play. Do you know how many three-point shots he's taken in his life? Do you know how many he's missed? I see guys who make themselves take two hundred shots before they allow themselves to leave the gym. Every day. After they're done with their workouts. Do you know how many times that natural messed up in a game? Made mistakes in other areas of his life?

The stumbles and the fumbles and the getting back up. The deep breath and the ability to take another shot. The willingness to throw up that three-pointer when it's the right shot at the right time, even though he missed his last four. That player can be proud in his success because he has earned every bit of it.

Look where you've worked hard and credit yourself.

TELL YOUR STORY

What are some of your accomplishments? Where have you worked the hardest in the past year? Decade?

Recall a specific moment when you stumbled or failed. Did you stay in the game? Did you make a strategic pivot? Did you get back up again? How do you feel about your ability to persevere?

Maybe you're reflecting on this prompt and you're thinking, *You know, Doc, I don't like to stick it out. When I fail, I tend to leave the court.* That's okay if that's how you've behaved until now, but next time I want to challenge you to stay in the game just for one more play. If you want to know a deep and abiding sense of pride, failure and persistence are going to be key to that experience.

Now that we've reflected more broadly, let's zoom in a little bit. Name three things you are proud of this past week. Something small, like showing up on time to your meetings, is fine. Saying "I love you" to your kids counts too.

What makes you feel most alive?

I t's probably not surprising that most of the players I work with say the basketball court is where they feel most alive. When they hear the ball bounce on the hardwood floor, everything sharpens. They are purely in the moment, in control. They get to be themselves here—no masks, no airs.

What makes me feel wide awake and alive? Resolution. Being able to resolve tension in my own life or someone else's gives me a feeling of accomplishment, a feeling of winning (and you know I like that). Feeling alive is not just some positive space. It's an energy, an adrenaline.

I was in Vegas with family, and we had a server who was in a bad mood. Some people at the table wanted to get into it and be edgy right back. But I reminded them we have no idea what the server's situation was—maybe someone in her life passed away or she's having trouble in a relationship. We needed to provide space and be gentle. And when we all made an effort to be gentle and nice, the server's approach quickly changed. The tension provided me with a chance to encourage resolution and peace, to employ my skill set that makes me feel alive.

What makes you feel alive? You can get clues by tuning in to your physiology throughout the day. When does your heart rate go up? When does your energy spike? When are you fired up? In the zone? Let's use the frame the players gave us too. When do you feel the most in control? The most focused? When do you get to truly be yourself?

Another way to think about when you are most alive is when you are most focused and in control. In these moments of peak energy, where do you naturally lock in, show up, and meet the moment?

And there's a flip piece to this, which is budgeting your energy. Pursuing those moments when you feel alive means you're going to need to reserve energy for them. They give us energy, but they demand it too. Recognize that energy is finite. Give a no without an excuse when needed. Hold that energy for other spaces.

Your time here on earth is limited, and it's your responsibility to find and do what makes you spark. Protect it, honor it, take joy in it. Live your life full of life.

TELL YOUR STORY

Throughout the day, take note of the times when you feel most energized. Take note of your physiology. Heart rate up, energy level up. You may discover something unexpected. Maybe you think of yourself as disorganized, and yet straightening up your desk gave you a boost. Who knows? Keep a list this week of small moments that feel heightened.

In your journal make a table with the hours of the day when you're awake, and then two columns for "Most Energized" and "Most in Control." Record the times of day when you are most focused and in control, two measures of feeling alive. What do you notice while looking over this record of peak energy and peak control? Do the two overlap? When?

Explore one activity or quality on this list with intentionality over the next month. Set a reminder on your calendar to check in and evaluate if this thing still sparks life in you. If so, create long-term strategies to continue incorporating this quality or activity into your life.

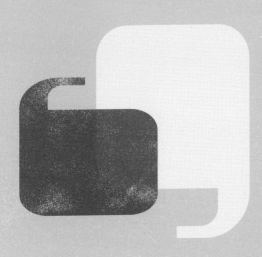

Your time here on earth
is limited, and it's your
responsibility to find and do
what makes you spark.

What are your values, and where did they come from?

If you followed me for a few days, you would see I have a pretty good rapport with the team's bus driver and the arena's janitor. I ask them how they're doing, if everything is good. "Most people don't talk with me," they say. The driver adds, "They just see me as the person driving the team from A to B." I don't operate that way. I want to create a trusting space with everyone. My dad taught me early on to be as kind to the janitor as I am to the CEO—or even kinder. That's a value I learned from him. I know exactly where it came from.

I've never been one who just follows the crowd. That's a value I got growing up Black in a mostly white town. "You're gonna stand out, bud. It's just what it is," my family told me. "You're gonna be the only Black kid in class, one of a few Black kids on sports teams. We're going to stand on who we know we are." My family instilled in me that integrity is a key part of the Yeager DNA. That's still true in our family today.

I knew when my parents were gone, it was dependent on me to carry their values forward. To move forward, a lot of times we need to reflect back. This is the African-based concept of *sankofa*. Always moving forward, yet also looking back. Take time to reflect back on the journey and the people who have helped to develop how you see the world. Parents, grandparents, neighbors, friends, romantic partners, classmates, coworkers—all these people have an influence on us.

Oftentimes, values can shift or change, or you may feel pulled in opposite directions. Maybe you go away to college with value systems you feel are pretty strong. Four years pass with people challenging some of those values, rigorous classroom discussions, new ideas and new insights, and those values may emerge with significant differences.

Given that you are evolving as a person, it makes sense that your values will evolve as well. When that happens, you might feel disloyal to the folks who handed you the value system. You don't want to reject the people who have shaped you. But your self-growth is not a criticism of anyone else. You can thank the people who taught you what they knew and welcome them to continue on a journey with you. This is sankofa. If they choose to stay behind, that's their choice.

As your values evolve or change, you may upset or

disappoint people. Not everyone is going to like it. You may not get the support you want. So you have to be strong in your new space, and you're going to have to fight some people to stay there. They may try to influence your values, just like they may have tried to author your story. I want to help you stay in the space of comfort with who you are and who you're becoming.

Values are not attained in a vacuum. All of us are formed by the people and places around us, much like a piece of clay. But unlike an inanimate piece of clay, we also bear responsibility for the values we hold. We are participants in our present and future selves. Gaining awareness of our value systems and where they come from gives us power to move forward into our futures with more clarity of what we want to change and what we want to keep. When it comes to value setting, awareness is your power, curiosity is your weapon, and your actions are the story the world will tell long after you're gone. This is your shot to write a story you're proud of.

TELL YOUR STORY

First, take an inventory of your values and how they were shaped. Consider what you observed or heard about money, spirituality, work, relationships, education, and the environment in your family of origin. Was your family emotionally open with one another? Did you integrate your everyday life with your neighbors? What was the most important character trait in the home you grew up in?

Each of these values has its own origin story. Choose one category listed above and track that value over the course of your life in five-year increments. Chart it on a graph if that makes sense to you. For every tick on the graph, mine your memory for a different story of how that particular value played out in your life. Write those stories. See what emotional experiences come up for you as you track this value through your life so far.

It's going to take a bit of time. Go on, I'll wait. It's worth it. Because in these stories you will find texture, nuance, and sometimes flat-out U-turns in your value systems.

Next, ask yourself, *Am I okay with my current value system? Do I want to change it? Do my actions align with the values I profess to hold?* For example, if you believe we should help those less fortunate, are you finding time in your schedule to lend a hand to others?

Draw a picture with yourself at the center. Then draw people who influenced your value system around you. Draw arrows showing the influence and add labels. Now draw a new version of you, away from the force of other people's influence. How does this person want to approach the world? Do you see any similarities between the two drawings? Differences?

Try to devote a little time this week to reading an article, watching someone on TV, or listening to someone speak with whom you disagree. For this exercise you needn't engage—in fact, it's better if you don't. Merely observe and listen. Give your curiosity muscle a workout. Why does that person think that way? What are her reasons? What evidence does she use to support her argument? When we are curious listeners, we have the opportunity to sharpen and shift the values we hold, while also gaining empathy for those who hold oppositional values.

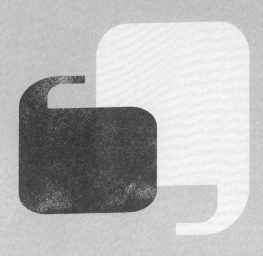

When it comes to value setting, awareness is your power, curiosity is your weapon, and your actions are the story the world will tell long after you're gone.

What are your nonnegotiables?

We develop nonnegotiables, what we must have in order to function and thrive, from experience. We are always learning. *This worked. This didn't.* When a relationship doesn't work out, we should take a moment to think about what wasn't right. That's good data to have going forward.

Start to be comfortable with owning your deal breakers. You'll save a lot of energy. Perhaps you try a long-distance relationship and realize it just doesn't cut it. You need to be in a relationship with someone you see most days in person. As you move forward and seek new relationships, you won't waste time with someone who is gone half of every month. When your new love interest says he's moving away to a different state, you know it won't work for you. It's nothing personal, but it is a deal breaker. Maybe it works fine for someone else. But you're not someone else.

A nonnegotiable has a finality to it, or at least a severity, but there can be flexibility in this space too. It can transition and shift. Based on a new life experience, maybe something you always thought was a nonnegotiable turns out not to be. But having them helps when you encounter someone and see what their limits are, so you know where yours are. Establishing non-negotiables is about setting the rules and making them clear. So there's an awareness piece with yourself, and then there's the communication piece when it comes to other people.

Communicating your nonnegotiables doesn't need to be a negative experience. It can be matter-of-fact. *Here are some things I really don't see changing in my life. Are you okay with that?* The other person doesn't have to be okay. But you have to let them know up front if something really is a deal breaker. A lot of people don't want to have those conversations. *If I say this, the relationship will unravel.* Better to know that now than years down the line, right?

One of the places nonnegotiables are most clear in my daily life is on the basketball court. There are different colors painted on the floor so you know what's in and what's out of bounds. *In* has no meaning without *out*. If you dribble the ball and it touches that line, you have to turn the ball over to the other team. Relationships are similar. There are areas that are out of bounds. Nonnegotiables aren't anything to be afraid of, because they define what is in bounds, the place where the relationship thrives. Don't think of boundaries with another person as being harsh or aloof. Think of them as being clear about the rules.

As you navigate these conversations, conflict will arise, but conflict is not a bad thing. You might see it as daunting, but conflict out in the open helps you seek resolution. If resolution can be found, then the relationship is healthy. Setting nonnegotiables helps you move the conflict outside yourself. That's where you can find resolution. Even if the resolution means saying goodbye. Saying goodbye now rather than five years from now is telling the truth.

Nonnegotiables and boundaries offer protection for yourself and your relationships. Consider how these might help your journey to discover how you are doing and how you could do better.

TELL YOUR STORY

When a friendship, work partnership, or romantic relationship hasn't worked well, what have been the primary areas of conflict?

What is out of bounds for you in a relationship? Could any of those nonnegotiables change in the future? What would the conditions have to be for them to change? Does that mean they weren't really nonnegotiables, or did you change?

Think of some areas in your life where you feel interpersonal tension. First, clarify where you feel the conflict is arising from. Are your nonnegotiables pulling in opposite directions? Consider the best possible setting to address this conflict, dependent upon the person.

The approach doesn't have to be aggressive. You can even ask for permission to challenge, something I do in therapy. Maybe it's a matter of asking, "Can I push back on some of the things you said recently?" As you talk, it helps to reiterate the other person's point through your conversation. Clarify throughout. "So, hold on. I heard you say this. I just want to be sure I caught what you said and that I'm getting it." Practicing your communication will help you establish and maintain your nonnegotiables.

What does living with intentionality look like for you?

Imagine you're at the free throw line and you've missed four baskets in a row. The ref hands you the ball and you miss a fifth. He hands it to you one more time. You pause. Take a step back. Take a deep breath. Reset. And now you step back up to the line with intention.

Living with intentionality doesn't have to be complex. It's really just acting consistently with your goals and your values, or as Henry David Thoreau called it, "living deliberately." [4] It involves knowing your whole being—your thoughts and your feelings—and moving purposefully toward your goals based on that.

It's easy to live in a reactionary space. Good things happen, and you start to think you're unstoppable. Bad things come, and you unravel. Daily life unfolds, and you respond. But hear me—*you have more power than that.* You can take control of a situation and think through how to respond. This is living with intention.

Instead of barreling through a presentation, take a few deep breaths before you begin. Look around. Marvel at the good fortune you have to share your knowledge. Smile at a few people in the audience. Be grateful that they're curious to hear what you have to say. And if things don't go perfectly, relax. You already made your shot by showing up with intentionality.

To put this into practice, I like to set aside time in the morning to evaluate the day before and think about the day ahead. Some days I'm relaxed and upbeat. *Hey, that was pretty good yesterday. I pulled that off.* And other days I have to be honest and realize I didn't follow through on my intentions the day before. *You were on some BS yesterday, Corey.* However the conversation goes, making time to think through the previous day helps with the day ahead.

For a lot of people, the biggest hurdle is finding the time. I'd like to encourage you to find an activity you absolutely can't miss and assign that time to be intentional *just about you.* For my youngest son, that intentional time is in the shower, since it's a daily activity he doesn't miss. He used to listen to music in the shower. I asked him to consider turning off the music and using that time to focus on how he might approach the day, to think, *How do I want to act today? What do I need to focus on?* He tried it and said he'd never turn on music in the shower again. (Not all my lessons stick that quickly.)

The pro basketball players I work with have similarly discovered a built-in time to be intentional. They stretch fifteen minutes every day, seven days a week. It's usually at the same time, which makes it even better. I often observe them while they're bending and reaching up, and I know they're mentally going to a different place. "I was rehearsing practice," they often tell me. Others focus on events later that day, mentally preparing for conversations and opportunities ahead. If this sounds like the visualization we already talked about, you're right. Intentionality is building on that practice.

Whenever possible, intentionally move with positivity. But realistically, not every day is a happy-face, giggly day and you'll want to tear some people up over things. An offensive move, when controlled and deliberate, can also be intentional. What you want here is for your intentions to be a reflection of your whole self—your purpose and your emotions. Living intentionally instead of reacting to whatever life throws your way will give you more control over your thoughts and feelings, helping you move toward goals with less stress.

TELL YOUR STORY

Think about your schedule for the next few days. Look for regular activities throughout the day when you could begin an intentional practice. Be creative. Can you think through your day while you're in the shower? On the train? On the treadmill? While making your morning coffee?

And don't stop with the scheduled moments of intention. Tune into the moments when you find yourself being reactionary. Take those moments as a cue that it's time to reset your power. What can you do that will reconnect you to your intention? We'll explore more techniques later. For now, take the first step to stop, take a breath, and focus yourself deliberately.

For five mornings in a row, when you wake up, ask yourself, *How do I want my day to go?* If you can, write down your intention for the day. It can be general: I will spread positivity. Or it can be specific: I will introduce myself to one new person. At the end of the five days, reflect back. Did setting that intention have any effect on the way you moved through the day?

Do you seek out laughter?

Recently a mother of two kids told me about her son's meltdown on a family trip. He became so distraught when he couldn't get the rental skates on his "enormous" feet that he ended up ditching the family and sulking around a state park by himself until it got dark enough and cold enough that he came back and found them. The mother had been annoyed with the scene and, before he took off, told her son he needed to deal with the discomfort of the skates and try to have fun. *Try to have fun.*

Did her reprimand relieve the tension? Not really. I had another idea. What if instead of pushing back and minimizing the issue, she had joined her son in his meltdown? She could have said, "These freakin' skates, they don't fit. This is total BS. Let's go up to the desk and let them know it's complete BS that they're trying to rent us these tiny skates." She could act out her son's anger—which is really about the discomfort of being an adolescent—and maybe helped him recognize the humor in the situation. At the very least he would have probably given the skates another try rather than let his mom continue to make her own scene.

We've all heard the saying, "Laughter is the best medicine." Well, it turns out there is science behind it. You actually take more oxygen into your lungs when you laugh. Laughter releases endorphins, reduces stress, and enhances your immune system. We might not all be comedic geniuses, but we all have the ability to be lighthearted. Tapping into that ability will improve our health, our mood, and even our communication skills.

When I meet a guard on the Pistons, I might start off by saying, "You ain't got no handles." (Translation: You can't dribble well.) The guard will look at me in confusion at first. He knows he is one of the best dribblers in the world. I smile and the confusion soon turns to laughter. He realizes I'm kidding around. That kidding opens the gates to the playground.

Laughter, jokes, silliness—they pull down the barriers between us. That's what I want to do in therapy. I want the walls to shrink away.

Laughter reassures us that things are going to be okay. If I'm about to be candid with someone about a tricky topic, I employ humor. Laughter helps us open space to acknowledge the deeper and harder things we've got going on.

Some of my players have gone through significant trauma in their lives. And especially in these conversations, I've found a good gut laugh to be healing. It signals, *It's gonna be okay. Something will come from this that will be all right.* That's the subtext. We're not saying it outright, but we're enacting it through our laughter. The lightheartedness does a lot of heavy lifting.

I choose to start every day with a bit of lightness. When I talk to the mirror in the morning, I smile and sing a little bit of Bill Withers's song "Lovely Day." I know I have that person in the mirror. I know that person has the ability to smile. It's going to end up being okay. This is what's worked for me. Maybe you can take this idea about laughter and find your own spin on it. Maybe you can tell me I ain't got no handles. (You'd be right.)

TELL YOUR STORY

Not only is laughter important in therapy and when engaging with others, but it's also a tool you can use on your own. What makes you laugh? It may seem like a trivial question at first, but it's actually profound. Are you laughing in your day? If not, can you start? Just like the linchpin challenge we talked about earlier, laughing can be the flip, a linchpin solution. Laugh more, and a lot of other pieces of your life will start to fall into place. Tension will lift. Work will go by faster (if you want it to).

What song can you sing in the morning to start your day with a smile? Start making a list of songs you hear that might work. As you hear songs in the days to come, think about how they make you feel.

What are some movies that make you laugh? TV shows or videos?

Are there times you could use humor strategically? Start paying attention to moments when it could be effective. If you are going to give a public speech, could you begin with a joke to put the audience at ease? If you're going to meet someone for the first time, can you make a self-deprecating comment to set a light tone? If you're working with someone who is upset, can you help them see the potential silliness in the situation?

Next time you feel aggravated, try to imagine your life from the outside as a blooper reel. I like to imagine I'm in an episode of *black-ish* or *Modern Family*. When we apply this frame, we realize most of our daily affronts aren't as serious as we think they are.

Who determines your joy?

In Minneapolis I helped create the Office of Black Male Student Achievement. We were focused on closing the perceived achievement gap for Black males. In that work I talked to students a lot about their academic struggles. Many told me their poor coursework had led to their parents feeling upset with them. Teachers were disappointed too. The classroom was devoid of hope. What usually helped turn things around was to take schoolwork little by little, assignment by assignment—to shift each student's mindset from disappointing others and toward the sacred practice of curiosity. Whatever the external factors, that internal curiosity was within their control.

"The grade is not what you're chasing," I told them. "You're chasing a deeper understanding of the material." This helped them become more internally driven. It was a process, but ultimately, most of them could see they wanted the ball in their court. They wanted the strength inside of them, in their control, not reflected in an abstract grade. Bring the ball into your court!

Get curious, and ask yourself what specific thing *inside your control* you can do today. For me—I seek to smile and be smiled upon every day. That's a pretty general goal, but it's also incredibly specific. It's achievable, measurable, and I know what I can do to influence the likelihood of reaching it. Even if I walk into really negative spaces today, I know I can smile. No one can take that from me. Some people are surprised that's all I want day to day, but you know what? My life is my court, and my days are determined by me. And I've decided I think a smile is pretty good.

Because the reality is, you're going to have to do some things in life that you don't look forward to. Maybe you hate your long commute. What are ways that you can control your happiness within this event? Maybe it's an opportunity for uninterrupted time to read or listen to a podcast. Any event that causes you anxiety is a chance for you to practice self-soothing strategies when they really matter. Sure, we can all feel at peace sipping iced tea on the beach in August, but when you're walking into a tough conversation with your boss on a dreary winter day? You're going to need some strategy to stay in control and not give in to the cynicism and ice.

And as it turns out, my smile works all year long.

TELL YOUR STORY

Whenever you can redirect your focus from your external circumstances to an internal place of control, you're bringing the ball into your court and are on your way to winning. Look at your calendar for the next week, and define the spaces that regularly bring you the most stress and negativity. Identify two to three strategies within your control to bring your values, humor, or genius into this space. Examples include:

- *For a standing meeting that regularly upsets you, choose to enter the room with the intent to ask questions.*
- *For those difficult hours putting your kids to sleep, think of a funny bedtime story you can tell, maybe even one about an exhausted, overwhelmed parent! Or flip your frame for how you'll use this time. Listen to some music or an audiobook that makes you feel alive.*
- *For when you're balancing your bank account, rather than approaching this space with judgment or spiraling fear, approach with a simple goal to gain clarity on your finances.*
- *For that dreaded grocery store trip, focus on the abundance available to you. For most of human history, and for many people around the world, the next meal is never a guarantee. Become curious about the food items and where they came from.*

You can also look for moments in your schedule where you can conserve energy for the things that really matter. How will you prioritize your day? Just like a power grid, you want to conserve and store energy for times of peak demand. Protect that inner you. Set yourself up to be better in control.

Pick one goal on the list for next year. It's likely that your goal will require some luck, the favor of others, or something else entirely outside of your control. That's life. But with every personal goal you have, there is always something you're responsible for. What does a win for one day look like? Do that one thing and be proud.

Who are the real models in your life?

T oo often we talk about having role models in our lives. But those are people with whom we'll never be able to engage. They're out there somewhere on the stage or at the stadium. In magazines or on our social media feed. Malcolm X is a role model for me. I admire that he was self-taught. MLK is a role model too. I especially admire the way they each behaved toward the end of their life. They both had to know that they most likely weren't going to be allowed to live. In the face of that existential threat, they both continued to press forward. They stayed the course. And what's more, they both continued to grow and learn and adopt new sensibilities until the end. They remained open, curious, and continually evolving in their thinking. MLK wondered if he had been too conciliatory. Malcolm realized not all whites were the enemy. The word *admire* is not deep or profound enough to describe how I feel about them.

These role models may inspire us, but it's important to have *real* models too. A real model is someone you can touch and be around. Someone with whom you can share the same space. Someone who can speak life into you. Someone who can call out your giftings. Someone who understands your values, so they can speak truth back to you.

My grandmother—everyone called her Granny Georgie, whether she was their grandmother or not—was a *mitzvah* in my world. She grew up in a family of sharecroppers in Mississippi. In the midst of Jim Crow, in flight from the KKK, her father made his way to Kansas, the first state where Jim Crow laws loosened up a little bit. Before long he sent for my grandmother, her siblings, and their mother, and together they settled three miles north of the Oklahoma border—far enough to escape the worst of persecution from the KKK. They were part of what's called the Great Migration. I don't see it as a migration, but more of a refugee movement.

My family grew up in the house next door. My grandparents were another set of parents to me and my siblings, always out in the garden and the yard, dropping little jewels of wisdom to everyone in the neighborhood.

Don't become someone your family won't recognize.

If you find success, remember the people who helped you get there.

And for me specifically: *As a Black man, people are going to put burdens on you. If there are burdens you can release on your own, do that—get 'em off you.*

From that last one I understood the importance of forgiving others. It was something I would have to do my whole life, and it was an unshackling, an unburdening. Our family—blood related or not—had no choice but to stick close together. There were so many forces against us, we would have been lost without that kinship.

At an early age I knew I noticed things other people didn't. I knew I had a lot I wanted to talk about, figure out, and discuss. More than most people around me. But not more than Granny Georgie. I watched people come to her for counsel on a weekly basis. They would play dominoes at a large table in her dining room while they talked. I don't know exactly what she said because she would tell the kids to get out of earshot.

But I knew people kept coming back for more of whatever advice she doled out. When I was ten, the age Granny Georgie had last had formal schooling, she took me aside and said, "I see something in you. It's what I have, the gift of discernment. Utilize it. Practice it. Watch people. Watch situations, and try to predict what will occur."

Granny Georgie shared her gift of discernment widely and freely. In fact, she shared everything she had with abandon.

She was a big piece of what held our collectivist community together. In her world, everyone was extended family. It's what we in the African American community commonly call "fictive kinships." Plus, my grandparents always had people living with them. My parents did, too, bringing in nieces and nephews to live with us. This is a generational pattern I've continued with my wife. I saw what my grandmother and mother did, and I wanted to do the same. Carrie and I brought in two young men to live in our home, and we're raising these adopted sons alongside our three biological boys.

My grandmother was a real model for me. We shared the same natural gifting, but I also got to see how she activated that gift for the goodness of everyone else. Not just for herself, but for the good of all of us. She was the wisest person I knew—and have ever known. I watched her for cues about how to move through life. "Move with wisdom, not knowledge," Granny Georgie would say. "Recognize the difference in knowledge and wisdom. Knowledge is information you can hold, and wisdom is the application thereof. It doesn't do us any good if we have knowledge but we're not applying it." We'd all do well to take a cue from Granny Georgie.

A role model helps you understand great things are possible. A real model helps you understand that great things are possible *for you.*

I got the idea of real models versus role models from Michael Walker, the director of the Office of Black Male

Student Achievement, whom I worked with in the Minneapolis Public Schools. A lot of the Black male students we worked with didn't have models for their everyday life. They needed to see us supporting them in the school setting. That was what had a powerful influence on them. (By the way, I was on Michael for three years to pursue his PhD. Now I'm on his dissertation committee.)

When my youngest son was ten, I pulled him aside and recreated the scene with Granny Georgie and me from back in Kansas. I told him I recognized in him the qualities of discernment and curiosity. Granny Georgie had recognized something in me that came to fruition decades later. Will my son one day tell a similar story? I try to be a real model for him the way Granny Georgie was for me. Living in her footsteps, carrying on her legacy. I take this role seriously, and I learned from the best.

TELL YOUR STORY

Who are your role models? What do you admire about them? Which of their attributes would you like to emulate?

Who are your *real* models? Who do you watch for cues about how you should act? Can you find any real models at work? Or in hobbies, at church, in your neighborhood? You don't have to admire everything about someone to appreciate certain qualities.

Pick one of the people you just listed, and let them know you consider them a real model. Name that goodness and call it out in the world, just like my Granny Georgie did for me! I'm convinced we don't do that enough. You have the power to encourage someone else, and invite them into this mentorship role in your life. As they've honored you with their talents and giftings, you can also honor them with your kind words.

Do you know what's behind your anger?

I got on a call the other day and found myself feeling a little on edge. Now, as a Black man in America, I don't have the privilege of showing that I'm on edge. This is one of the many jewels of wisdom Granny Georgie passed along to me. Showing that I'm on edge could threaten my life. But I felt my heart rate increase, my mouth become dry, a wave of heat pass over me. A few minutes in, I recognized that I needed to stop talking. I knew my anger was masking something else.

I'd been doing some work with myself in front of the mirror and thinking about loneliness. At the time I'd been staying in Detroit with the Pistons, away from my wife and kids. I love working with the guys. I feel joy in that. But in the afternoons after practice, I typically drive to my apartment and know I won't engage face-to-face with another person until the next morning.

At first I didn't think of this situation as problematic. I love my job. I like spending time with myself. I know my wife has everything handled at home. But something started bubbling up. So I had to sit with myself, look at myself in the mirror, turn off the music, turn off the media, and think, *What am I feeling?* The best description I could think of was *lonely*. I felt lonely, maybe for the first time in my life.

On that phone call, I was able to direct myself into silence. I stopped talking, reminding myself of my earlier conversation with myself, and said—*that's loneliness*. I was able to bring the true feeling forward into consciousness. That's powerful, because doing so can stop me from entering a tense conversation or even an argument. I don't have to tell the other person what's going on. I can choose to share that information or not. I might even end the call with, "Hey, this isn't the best time for me to talk. Can we talk tomorrow?" But I had *access* to the truth of what was going on. And from that awareness, I could move with intention.

I have players who sometimes present with anger. I move quickly to curiosity about the root of that anger because I know it's often a secondary emotion. "I hear you're pissed. Is that anger because you're disappointed in yourself? Is it because you're sad about something?" They don't always go with me immediately, but if we sit with it a little, we often find something. "I'm upset that I busted my butt and didn't get the result I wanted."

Once we get to the root of the anger, then we're able to play with that primal emotion. Now we're in the playground. Or maybe the battlefield. I find anger often masks disappointment and sadness—two emotions that are hard to discuss. For many of us, it's easy to talk about being angry. Fuming. Wanting to punch the wall. But anger doesn't come out of nowhere. Scratch the surface a bit and you'll often find some variation of sadness.

Being angry in certain situations is natural, and it can be an appropriate and healthy response to many situations. In my role as a therapist I normalize that emotion. Your suffering is not unique. Many others are having the same struggle. But where did this anger come from? We have to get to the sadness and disappointment underneath it. But then the question becomes, What are you supposed to do with this heavy anvil that is drowning your soul?

My wife is Jewish. Being around her family I've learned the custom of sitting *shiva*, sitting with mourners in their intense period of grief. It's not about having answers. It's not about affirming. It's about community, presence. It's just about being, which is one of the greatest gifts we have to offer. I'm here, and I'm going to stay here. I am continuously sitting shiva for the grief and loss of people and relationships, and the grief and loss of the old versions of ourselves we're now outgrowing.

As a therapist my first priority is to be with you and give

you my presence. Oftentimes, that's all you are looking for. In your overwhelming sadness, the most comfort you can have is often the true, unshakeable presence of someone else. If you have someone who can give you that, grab hold of it with all your might.

TELL YOUR STORY

When you start to feel tension, an increased heart rate, and other signs of agitation, try to pause and pull back from the situation. Can you have a quick conversation with yourself? What are you feeling? Why might you be feeling this way? Could another feeling be underneath?

If you experience anger as a prevailing emotion, I'd challenge you to start writing about those moments or recording them in a voice memo. See if there's a common theme or motif in those stories. This will help you identify the root of your anger. We're always interested in root systems, because when we get down there and start digging out the source, we have better clarity and control.

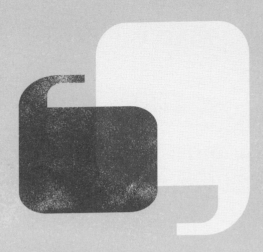

I find anger often masks
disappointment and sadness—
two emotions that are hard
to discuss.

What do you most hope to accomplish in your future?

Every day, I'm surrounded by guys who are at the pinnacle of the sport. They got to the top of their Everest. But what happens when you get to the top? Sure, you've got a great view, but the journey can't end there. And it doesn't. Some want to become a starter. Others talk about winning championships. But even with their sights set ahead, they appreciate the reminder to keep dreaming. We all think about our future and what's next.

When the late Kobe Bryant retired from the LA Lakers in 2016, he was widely acknowledged as one of the greatest basketball players of all time. In addition to pro ball, he became a producer and a writer, winning an Oscar for his short film. He wanted to be the best in those fields too. Even though he was at the top of one mountain, he was always moving forward, setting new goals.

A competitive nature can drive us forward. I have one. When someone tells me I'm dreaming too big, that adds forty horsepower to my engine. There were plenty of naysayers around when I was pursuing my PhD. The naysaying motivated me. *Let's see what you say when I walk the stage and they hand me that degree,* said my internal voice. I knew part of the doctoral process was to weed people out. About 40 percent of my cohort made it; 60 percent fell off. I was the first Black male in twenty-six years to finish the PhD in my department. I was an anomaly, a unicorn. *Tell me I can't do something, I'll show you I can.* In those years, I drew on some advice from my father. He said I didn't have to tell people what I was about. I would just show them. Anybody can talk about climbing their Mount Everest, but it's a whole lot more impressive if you actually do it.

And I did.

And I'm proud.

That kind of joyful pride is available to you too. When you think about what you most want to accomplish in your future and how you're going to get there, keep in mind that essential, original question—*Who is the most important person in your life?* What are the dreams you have for yourself? Are you stuck on an old dream or in need of a new one? Maybe it's time to aim higher, move forward, or set new goals.

Carve out some precious time to dream—really dream, like you're a kid again. And then listen to the words of my dad. *Just show them.* Remember the elephant?

Take small bites. Start eating.

TELL YOUR STORY

What do you hope to accomplish? Make a list of ten goals, big and small. Pick one, and put it on the far right side of the page. This is the finish line. Now go back to the left side of the page and write "START." What are the in-between steps you need to take to get to the finish line?

For example, let's say you want to own a house. First you have to improve your credit score. To do that, what are the first bills you're going to pay off? Paying those bills is bringing you closer to the dream of the house. You pay those bills, your credit score rises, you get approved for the loan, you find a house that works for your family, you sign the paperwork, and you see your wife's face as the Realtor hands her the keys.

Moving from the dream to reality has all these steps in between, and some may cause friction. The dream inspires you, but the bills won't pay themselves. The dream can be humungous, but the steps to get you there are generally small. You don't have to shrink the dream, but the steps have to be rooted in reality.

Are you driven by the desire to prove yourself? What other forces motivate you? Once you define those forces, it's important to saturate your daily life with them. Name a few spaces and people who bring out the dreamer in you. Now name a few folks who will hold you accountable to that dream. Consider giving them a call. No one gets to the top of Everest without a guide.

What do you most hope to change in your life?

One thing that can help us as we continue to grow is learning to make distinctions about change. There are different areas of our lives we want to change, but the *depth* of change also varies.

On one end of the scale you have minor changes, like removing sugar from your diet, and then there are major transformations, like switching careers. Which kind of change are you seeking right now—small or big, a reset or a revolution?

In couples therapy, we have a treatment called discernment counseling. Discernment counseling is a brief therapy where we help the couple decide what kind of change they're seeking. *What are we trying to do here? Are we going to work through this therapeutically, or are we going to help you separate your lives?*

It's a huge question, but it is still pre-therapy. Answering questions about what kind of change is needed and wanted helps us know what we are going to do in therapy, how the couple is going to move forward.

Applying this principle to your own life, whatever the area, before you begin changing, you have to figure out what kind of change you are seeking. Is it first order, like a couple making an effort to communicate better? Or is it second order, like a couple figuring out how to say goodbye?

I like to think of first- and second-order change in terms of home renovation. Taking the pictures off your wall would be a first-order change. Second order would be knocking a wall down, actually changing the structure of the home.

In your life right now, are you picking out paint colors or hauling out the sledgehammer?

Of course, it's easy to see the difference between first- and second-order change when we think of a home renovation, but it can be incredibly difficult to decide what kind of change you want. In some cases, you will know right away. Other times it's going to take reflection. Patience. Visualization. Imagination. Deep dives into the playground of your mind. Your desires and values may be at odds. You may have to battle it out. Many of the concepts we've been defining and practicing over the course of the book will come into play.

If you do determine you need second-order change, take a breath. No need to rush. No need to panic. As my mother would say, "It was the same length before you realized how far you had to go." What you've got now is an awareness of where to go. Now you can figure out how to get from here to there.

If you're met with resistance to your second-order change, don't be surprised. Friends and family may bristle at the changes you're making, especially if your life choices have a direct impact on them. But as you knock down the walls in your life, it's important to remember the deep work you did at the outset, and you owe it to yourself to honor your decision. Stay the course. Stay curious, stay kind, and trust that resiliency will follow.

TELL YOUR STORY

What obstacles are in front of you that require a change? Are they first-order or second-order problems? If you're having a hard time categorizing this, think about whether the change you desire will have a large ripple effect in your life. If so, this is likely a second-order change.

Pick one thing you want to change. Let's say you want to improve your ability to say no or to develop your nonnegotiables. You might think of this as a first-order change. After all, saying no is simply using a word more often. And maybe that's all it is—just brushing up on some self-protection skills.

But maybe you're finding there's a deeply rooted element to your inability to say no. Maybe you're experiencing a physiological change at the very thought of it. You might be looking at a second-order change. That's a good indicator that you're going to need to knock down some bigger untruths in your life, or start to have a conversation with yourself about your value system. This may be less about boundary setting and more about your desire to seek approval from others. Sheer willpower won't change that. Get in front of the mirror and gently ask yourself more questions about the untruths you're telling yourself.

What do you love most about being you?

My older brother was greedy when we were little. If we were having cake at a party, he would put the two pieces we were given side by side and compare them. The one with a little bit more icing, that's the one he would take. He was always comparing and always choosing the biggest and best version of everything for himself. I hated watching that greediness, and a deep sense of disgust toward greed took root in my childhood. I told myself I was going to be the opposite. I was going to give the cake with the most icing away to the next person. I would hang back and let others pick first.

The example of my brother's greed produced a generosity in me that I love about myself. In fact, I teach this kind of selfless, others-focused behavior to my sons. Something good grew out of something ugly.

This conversation continues our self-inventory work, and it is connected to the question of pride. What do we love about ourselves? Are we curious? Generous? Fair-minded? Hardworking? Adventurous? Patient? Spontaneous? And of course I'm not going to let you simply pick a few adjectives and go on to the next question. I want you to share your stories behind what you love about yourself, to find the origin points of what makes you *you*. I am always seeking stories because we need to string them together on our map to make sense of where we came from and where we're going.

Writing down those stories is also about becoming grateful for the life experiences—good and bad—that made you who you are. Yeah, I wish I had more chocolate cake growing up, but in my reflective time, I'm able to look back at those exchanges with my brother, and I'm thankful for them.

I'm not asking you to force gratitude where it's not available to you—I'm aware you've probably experienced something much harsher than being shortchanged some chocolate icing. But, as you're able, it's important to craft gratitude for the full array of experiences that have shaped you into the person you love. When you understand growth through the lens of gratitude, you'll be able to accept fearful or uncomfortable moments more readily. You never know what life experience could come around the corner that will shift you into someone you may love even more.

TELL YOUR STORY

If you're having trouble thinking about what you love most about being you, think about what you love in other individuals. Pick someone you adore. What do you love about him or her? What attracts you? What do you admire? This might produce the same answer for you or give you more insight into yourself coming from a different angle. You might have initially loved someone's boundless energy and now you admire how much they accomplish with that energy.

Now try the exercise again with someone who is quite different from the first person you picked. What do you love about this person? What qualities stand out? How does he or she light up the world?

You've done some warm-ups. You're starting to think about all the positives around you. Now let's look at you. What do you love about *yourself*?

How can you bring that quality to the spaces you are in? How can you not only author your own story but also change the bigger picture you are in? Are you bringing those qualities you love about yourself to the room, or are you holding back?

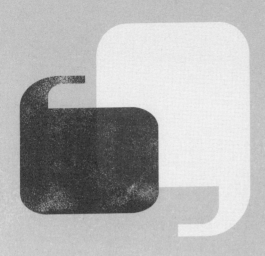

You never know what life experience could come around the corner that will shift you into someone you may love even more.

If you could change one experience in your past, what would it be and why?

When I talked earlier about my sacred spaces, there was one I didn't include. The place where I conjure up my father. Why did I hesitate to include that one? Maybe it felt too vulnerable at first. Maybe it felt silly or mystical. I can't stretch my dad's life past the time he had on earth, but there's something I can do. I can close my eyes and remember his laugh. If it's really quiet, and I'm home by myself on my favorite chair, I can almost hear his voice. I like to imagine advice he'd give me today if he were here. But I'm older than he was when he moved on. I've already had more years.

If I could change one thing in my life, I would have my dad stay alive for a longer stretch. I had him for fifteen years. If I'd had him longer, I would have made different decisions about where I played football. I know I would have graduated the first time I went to college because he would have stayed on me. I don't get to change the time my dad was here on earth, but it helps me to know that's what I would change if I could. It brings my life into sharper relief. It helps me know what is at the center.

What if Dad could have spent time with my kids? How would that have impacted them? What if he had smiled at my wife and made her feel loved? Would that change the relationship I have with her now?

We all have tons of things we might change. The task here is to prioritize. To make tough decisions, even just in the hypothetical. This calls on our powers of visualization from earlier in the book, but now we're going in a different direction. We're not visualizing what may be, but rather what could have been—in order to understand ourselves more.

You can interpret this question in different ways. Maybe you want to think about a decision you would make differently. Or a person you wish hadn't come into your life. Or hadn't left.

How do you go back to this experience but take care not to get lost there? How do you not live in regret? The key is to remember all of the experiences you've had that made you who you are. Let the people and places and regrets and sorrow that live on in your memory stir you to become a better you. Because you are still writing your story. Don't relinquish your pen to chapters that are closed. Pick it up, and write the ending you want to see.

The memory of my dad stirs me to become a better father. And hey, let's be honest, that's not always so easy. For instance, my sons used to bicker with each other. That was just their relationship. The rest of us were used to it and did our best to block out the noise. But one day when they were teens, I stopped their argument, sat them down, and had a conversation. "There's six hundred and some days before one of you goes off to college," I told them. "You have to get your relationship right now."

I lost my dad because of circumstances I couldn't control. I wasn't about to allow my sons to lose each other when they didn't have to.

"It's too late," they both said. The one thing they agreed on. But that wasn't true. They still had time living under the same roof, and they still had (and have) the rest of their lives. Today they're super close and they can laugh about what they used to argue about. They can't go back and change all those years of arguing, but they don't need to. They realized, *Hey, if I could change something, it would be to get along better with my brother.* And I think my dad would have liked to see them like this.

Today is a new day. What do you still have the power to change? Seize those places where you have agency. *It's set in stone,* we like to say. *It can't be undone. There's nothing I can do. It's in the past.*

Sometimes, yes. And to that, all I can say is I'm sorry. But don't let your mind become so obsessed with replaying pain that you refuse to stay present in your body. Don't let your losses tell you the lie that your smile will never come again. Honor the people, places, and dreams that you've lost with the promise to yourself that you will live in truth. In power. In agency. In love.

There's no better way to serve them. I promise you.

TELL YOUR STORY

If you got one shot to change the plotline that already played out, what would you change? Choose something. What would have gone differently? Go into your imaginative space.

Try to identify the latent value undergirding that experience. In losing my father, I recognized the primacy of familial love. That was my value I have sworn to uphold. What are the values you will champion to honor your past?

Write a letter to your former self. If you need to, extend grace, warmth, or forgiveness. Thank them for enduring this hardship. Let them know how you have grown and changed. Let them know it gets better.

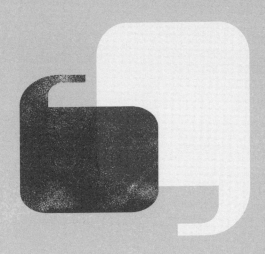

Today is a new day. What do you still have the power to change?

What healing do you seek in your life?

If you have an infection, a doctor can clean out the infected area and provide medicine. But there's one thing they can't actually do. They can't heal you. Your body has to do that work.

My healing has to come from me. Yours has to come from you.

The same is true in therapy. The therapist can guide you, but you have to do the work.

I once had a player who was new to the team. I was doing an initial interview like I do with all the players. This particular player began talking about his upbringing, including some traumatic experiences and the murder of loved ones. He was twenty-three. He'd made it to the NBA, a dream he'd had since he was seven. But he was still dealing with things many people won't face in their lifetimes. He had bottled up those memories. He told me he had never discussed them at all. That vulnerability, he reasoned, wouldn't help him in his journey to the NBA. "I've never cried about this," he told me. "I put it to the side and used it to motivate me."

This player was taught that vulnerability would hurt him, but in reality, by keeping these events below a conscious level of awareness, he was actually hindering his development. If you go through a traumatic experience, elements of your development are arrested at that age when it happened. It is crucial that you take the brave step to bring the trauma up to the surface, for your own good.

Relieve the pressure. That's what we're looking for when we're unpacking trauma. You can't undo the events of your past, but that deep intensity pressurized below the surface is a dangerous thing. The truth must be brought up to the surface, or it will continue to fester in your soul and your physical body.

But hear me that healing is possible. Trauma isn't going to heal overnight, but you are worth the long-haul process of becoming healthy. Maybe this book is enough to start bringing your trauma to the surface, but it's possible you'll need an assist from a therapist. Someone you can talk it out with. If you feel that impulse, I'd encourage you to try therapy out. You are worth growing up and out of what happened to you. No matter your story, no matter your past, you deserve to be in the playground.

What do you seek to heal? There are people out there who can help you with the process. You can get treatment. We all need some version of healing.

Do you know what areas of expertise you're looking for? Some therapists are great with grief and loss; others are great with anxiety. Some focus on career work. Others specialize in anger management. You can find ones who help with men's issues, women's issues, LGBTQIA+, relationships, PTSD. Find someone who has expertise in an area that's important to you. Sit with them. It's important for you to evaluate the fit. Does this person understand you? Can this person help you? You should be comfortable saying a person is not a fit. It's not a strike against that person; it's just not a match for you.

When my wife and I were preparing for our wedding, we had a bunch of different food tastings. When a food sample wasn't quite right, that wasn't a strike on the chef. It just wasn't our thing. There's no reason to worry about hurting someone's feelings if you choose not to work with that person. Someone might make the world's best bruschetta, but it just wasn't what you pictured for your buffet table. The best therapist is the one who works for you.

If you think you might want to engage a therapist, but you feel apprehension about taking the next step, why do you think that might be?

Don't get discouraged about this process of finding the right fit therapeutically. When you start paying attention to what needs to heal, you start the healing process. But remember, whether you're looking for guidance from a therapist or moving ahead alone, healing can only come from within.

What mistake have you learned the most from in your life?

Coaches review mistakes after a game to learn. The key words are "after a game." *During* the game you have to focus on the moment at hand. Players often have what I call *athletic amnesia*. Sometimes they want to temporarily forget—or block out—both the bad *and* the good. If they had a really great play, it doesn't serve them to be thinking about how good that play was as they move in to the next one. Same with a mess-up or mistake. Most players forget it in the current moment. The game is still unfolding, and timing is everything.

But when the time is right, we all need to know how to take on the role of "coach" and reflect on the mistakes we've made.

If you lost your temper one evening, you might be upset and regret your behavior. The adult thing to do is to accept the mistake, apologize, and promise to do better next time. But those moves alone don't necessarily set you up for a better next time. You need to dig into the roots of what went wrong. Maybe you skipped the time in the morning when you let yourself be intentional and visualize the day ahead. Without that time, it's hard to stay mindful. Did you start the day with intention? Did you put yourself first? Are you trying to steer your internal voice toward positive self-talk? Are you attacking the elephant of your challenges bite by bite? A misstep or two earlier on in the day can spiral so that by the time dinner rolls around, you don't have the restraint to hold your temper. Let's review the game play not only at that moment but also in the ones that led up to it. The passes, the blocks, the fumbles, the crossovers.

Your first step is to tell the truth. This is what happened. This is what you did. Many avoid that step, so if you're there with me telling the truth, good work.

Next is understanding. Why did that happen?

Next comes forgiveness. Forgiveness is the root of grace. I can't give grace to myself without first forgiving myself. That, too, is a critical piece. And once you're there, you can produce grace for yourself and others. Depending on the situation, you may need to apologize to someone else, but you have to get to the point where it's genuine before you do it. It could take two days or two years. You need to understand what you did wrong.

That may necessitate some conversations in the mirror. And when you do apologize, you cannot control whether you're forgiven by someone else. But you're unburdening yourself.

And sometimes there is even gratitude. If you had not made that mistake, you would not have learned this particular lesson. I welcome stumbles, because I love learning, and the mess-ups are where the best learning happens. If you never stumble, you aren't really challenging yourself. Plus, getting back up after a fall is a great lesson to pass onto others.

The most impressive growth happens in failure. As Nelson Mandela said, "I never lose. I either win or I learn." The mistakes you've made aren't about failing yourself. They're about finding yourself. When you stumble, you have the chance to learn. But learning can be uncomfortable. Pain means you're morphing into something new. You will still be uncomfortable, but remembering that the pain is an indication of growth lessens the sharpness of that pain.

TELL YOUR STORY

We've all made a zillion mistakes, some of them real doozies. So, let's prioritize. Let's warm up by looking at some small mistakes first and then at the roots that led to those mistakes. We're starting with a weight we can handle; we're training. We're learning the process of awareness and truth and forgiveness and grace. And one day, we'll be ready for the doozies.

Make a list of some recent actions you regret. What was your mind-set when you took that action? What circumstances led up to it? You may be in a similar situation moving forward and you will have a lot of data to draw on next time to make better decisions.

Consider if your mistake affected someone else. Do you need to ask for forgiveness for any of these recent actions? This is the time to engage with yourself—in the mirror, in your journal, in your chair beside the wolf painting—and think about what took place. What could you have done differently? Take the time you need to get to a genuine place of remorse before you approach someone to ask for their forgiveness. When you're ready, know you can only control your actions. What the other person says or does in response to your apology is beyond your control.

Do you love to win or hate to lose?

I don't think it's any secret by now that I love to win. The roar of the crowd when I used to rush the ball down the field, the adrenaline high on the sidelines encouraging my players, the feeling like you're floating on air, the camaraderie among the winning team—it can't be beat. It's exhilarating. You put all this energy and work into something and you came out victorious. Any win I'm part of seems to lift the energy of everyone around me. For all these reasons, I love to win.

I started to notice patterns with my players. More than loving to win, some hated to lose—they wanted to avoid the negative feeling that comes with losing. Others loved to win and they were seeking out that high. The love and the hate seemed to align with whether the players were optimistic, expecting good things—or pessimistic, worried about bad things happening.

I asked one player if he always hated to lose. He dug deep right away, reflecting back on a time when he was seven years old. It was the first time he remembers being responsible for losing a game. On the car ride home, his father was all over him. "You can't be a loser." From that moment on, he hated to lose, and that motivated him.

Another player remembered playing a game when he was around seven years old, and when his team won, everyone went to celebrate at his favorite restaurant. His mom and dad were laughing. His siblings and friends were all having a great time, his parents were giggling. It's a memory that stands out. He's always seeking that exhilarating feeling.

Do you love to win or hate to lose? Sometimes this question alone can give us insight into our personal history and our psyche. Do you want people to congratulate you, or are you more focused on avoiding disapproval? Do you want to turn in the best report in your department, or do you want to make sure you don't leave any room for criticism? Are you looking to get promoted or to avoid getting fired?

Loving to win is an affirming space. You're seeking positivity. You may also lean toward perfectionism. Those who hate to lose tend to be strong protectors, but they may lean toward negativity.

Loving to win and hating to lose might both lead to the

same outcome. But not always. At the extremes of each, they wrap around opposite corners and meet on the other side. But hating to lose might mean many different things. It might mean you don't ever want to be seen as weak or incompetent. That may lead to playing it safe, passing the ball when you're two points down with five seconds left in the game. Your teammate will have time to hurl up a two-pointer. But you had a chance to go for three. It was the right play, but looking back you might regret it.

Remember, it's about awareness, not being right or wrong. Are you aware of how you see the world?

TELL YOUR STORY

Do you love to win? What are the origins of that love? Or do you hate to lose? Where do you think that began?

Think of someone close to you who seems to have the opposite approach when it comes to winning and losing. Do you come into conflict over these differing perspectives? Does the love to win/hate to lose frame help you understand the other person's choices and behaviors any better?

Can you take the love to win/hate to lose frame and apply it to areas that don't have traditional winners or losers? For example, on a vacation, do you tend to seek out peak experience and adventure, or are you more tuned into making sure things don't go wrong, making dinner reservations, getting the group to the train station on time? Does the frame work in other areas? Does it help clarify different approaches that sometimes come into conflict?

What are the generational trends that pervade your family story?

In earlier chapters, I talked about the kinship community my parents and grandparents created when I was growing up in Kansas. That included welcoming in friends as family to our BBQs and even taking family members into the home. I brought that model to the family Carrie and I created. Mike is a friend of mine, but my boys call him Uncle. My wife's brother is also Mike, so the kids have two Uncle Mikes—one blood-related and one not. They don't distinguish between them. Carrie and I welcomed two young men into our home and we're raising them alongside our biological sons. This was the model I had growing up, and it's one I want to replicate.

But there was another generational pattern I wanted to change. In my family growing up, no one said the words "I love you." I knew my parents and grandparents loved me, but it wasn't out in the open. Hearing those words would have been affirming. Carrie grew up with a similar pattern. When we started dating we began to discuss this absence. In a way, we were looking back at the sixteen-year-old versions of ourselves. We wanted those kids to have the sense that saying "I love you" is the norm. Well, we can take action in the present, not the past. So we began saying "I love you" all the time to our boys, and they say it too. My sons can be in the living room and when they head upstairs to do homework, they call out, "I love you." The other night the younger one was taking about five steps away from where Carrie and I were sitting. "I love you," he called out over his shoulder.

This question about generational trends can help us stand back a bit from our lives and look at the family as a system. The first step is awareness. What are the trends we've been handed? The next step is a decision point. This is where you have control. How do you want to lead your life? Do you want to break patterns or replicate them?

Thinking and talking about our families can stir up deep feelings of nostalgia. A feeling of warmth that you long to replicate in relationships moving forward. For others, that's a door you want to seal shut forever. For most people, it's complex—a mix of both of those feelings. Notice where you are on that spectrum, even as different family members or patterns of behavior come to mind.

Remember that even as you reflect back, you're always moving forward. You can't change the past, but it provides you the wealth of knowledge you need to come into alignment with who you want to be. Some keys you need to unlock your present may be in these memories.

TELL YOUR STORY

Can you identify an emotional pattern in your family you'd like to keep? First, make a list of things you liked in your house growing up. Were birthdays special? Did you have an intentional morning or evening routine? Was there a particular way you celebrated a holiday? Was there any special family mantra or quirk that brings a smile to your face? How will you bring this pattern into your life today and going forward?

Now, without thinking too much about it, generate a list of things you wish you'd had more or less of as a kid. Do you wish conflict could have been out in the open instead of bubbling and brewing, with everyone dancing around it? Or do you wish there'd been a little more restraint, fewer tense discussions? Do you wish there'd been more time together as a family or that solitary time and solo pursuits had been encouraged?

Looking at this list, pick one item and decide how you're going to change the pattern going forward. What action can you take today to start a new pattern?

What can you do in twenty-three seconds?

I n basketball, a player who gets fouled gets a free throw. In between the foul call and the throw, he's got twenty-three seconds. I asked one of my players, "What do you normally do in that twenty-three seconds?" He stared back blankly.

That response helped us come to an awareness. His twenty-three seconds weren't being used. He gave that time away. What if he approached it differently? What if he said he was going to be intentional with even that little fraction of time?

A reduced heart rate gives players a better shot at making a basket. So in practice we did a test. A player got his heart rate up to 160 beats per minute on a stair-stepper. Then I gave him twenty-three seconds to bring down his heart rate. With some mindful breathing, he brought it down to the 140s. He was in a much better zone for making a free throw. All it took was an intentional use of that twenty-three seconds. That's how much control we have!

That player took this knowledge to the game. Now, after a foul, he is intentional about utilizing those precious twenty-three seconds to bring down his heart rate and center himself.

If NBA players can use twenty-three seconds effectively under that kind of pressure, I know you can effectively use little moments throughout your day. And guess what? No one else has to know you're doing it. Maybe before a meeting or an important phone call you can settle yourself, check in. Instead of scrolling mindlessly, be mindful about your next meeting or task. Instead of checking your texts in the three minutes before the kids get home, take some deep breaths and be fully present when they burst in the door.

This twenty-three-second framework is a fun and challenging way to think about how much you can accomplish in a small fraction of time. When I realized that some of the basketball players had developed an ability to center themselves on the go, it reminded me what incredible power we have, moment by moment, to ride the waves of all that life is going to bring our way. Even when you aren't able to slip away to spend time engaging yourself in the mirror—maybe you're midmeeting or at a tense dinner—you still have access to your intentionality. You can always stop to refocus, get a pulse on how you are and where you are, and bring that heart rate down—in almost no time at all.

All it takes is twenty-three seconds.

TELL YOUR STORY

First, take note of your mood at the current moment. Write a sentence or two about it. Time yourself for twenty-three seconds. Simply breathe deeply. Notice how your breath moves throughout your body. As your attention wanders, invite your focus back to your breath. Stop the clock and notice whether your mood has changed at all.

Look for micro-mindful moments throughout your day, times when you can take a breath and re-center. Now start tracking when you were successful re-centering yourself and when you couldn't bring your heart rate down.

If you'd like, get more specific in your record-keeping, noting date, time, location, and other important variables. Look for patterns. Are you better able to re-center in the morning than at night? Do you have trouble re-centering when you're in public? Does the presence of certain individuals or certain tasks make you particularly tense? If nothing else, perhaps you'll get guidance as to where you need the most practice, or a relationship you need to repair, or a deeper value system you need to spend more time with in the mirror. Remember, every time you go through the steps—deep breathing, maybe saying your mantra—you are practicing, whether you reach your goal of re-centering or not. I've seen many practices in my day. Whether you call them touchdowns, points, baskets, hits, or goals, sometimes hours and hours go by without reaching a single one. You put in your time on the field. That's all you can do.

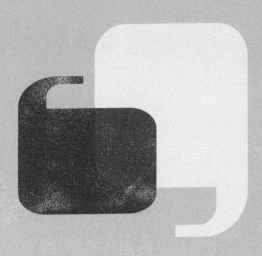

Today is a new day. What do you still have the power to change?

Are you coachable?

My parents and grandparents would have told you I was always asking questions. Sometimes it got me into trouble. I enjoyed studying calculus in high school, but I had a lot going on with football and friends, and I was puzzled as to the differential equation end game. One day I raised my hand. "I love how you teach," I told Mr. Harper. "But how will this help me when I'm forty? Can you help connect the dots?" I wasn't being critical; I was just curious. I thought I was opening a conversation where I would learn something not just about parabolas but about adulthood and what it entailed as well. Mr. Harper was not amused. In fact, he got mad. His anger stifled my curiosity for a period of time.

Fortunately, it didn't shut me down. Something told me I could stay curious, but what I had to be better at learning was when to *convey* that curiosity, especially with those who were in positions of authority and might feel threatened. From that interaction with Mr. Harper, I began learning how to maneuver. I could be curious, but I shouldn't ask a question like that in front of a class and appear disrespectful. I had to be aware of context and what makes people put their guard up. Calculus is the study of constant change; it's a study I've since devoted my life to, using different language.

The theme I want to highlight here, more than curiosity, is adaptability. Learning to pivot. I could have said to myself, *Hey, curiosity doesn't get rewarded—maybe I should ditch it.* But instead I found a better way to wield that curiosity. Like many gifts, it could serve me, but only if I knew how to use it properly.

In college football, I was what the coaches called a "highly coachable player." Later, in my doctoral program, I became a highly trainable doctoral student, always eager for advice. I take in feedback, even when it comes indirectly, like the calculus teacher bristling at my comment. I find a way to use that new information.

Let's look at this quality on a micro level. Many of us tend to react defensively when someone challenges us in conversation. We feel shaky and double down on our point. We scramble for evidence supporting why we are correct and why the other person is wrong. Or we change the subject.

How about becoming curious instead? Why not learn

something? "I never thought of that," you can always tell people, when it's true. You don't have to apologize. We all have different experiences, a variety of research we've done, unique ways of approaching problems. There are so many ways to look at the world. Why not appreciate a new angle?

My favorite moments in conversation are the break-throughs when, together, we discover something new. They're most likely to happen when people bring different perspectives to the conversation. That's when you get synergy, something greater than each person would have created alone. This connects back to learning from each other, and *with* each other.

If you go through life without asking questions or taking in feedback, it means you have to think of everything on your own. It means you can never make a mistake (good luck with that). It means if you get new information that's inconsistent with your theory, you have to refute it, discard it, belittle it, and be defensive about it. And it also means you won't grow from that new data. Relax. Listen. Even if you are the smartest person in the room, you can't see behind your own back, so listen to the guy who can. Maybe that person knows something important. And it's easier than continually spinning around to try to see everything at once.

This partly comes down to role clarity. If I'm the center on the basketball team, my job is not to bring the ball up the court. It will get stolen, and I would be costing the team. We play as a team, but we each have to play our individual parts.

In football, an offensive lineman's job is to block. They have to focus on keeping guys off the quarterback so he can throw and open up lanes to run with the ball. These are supportive roles. One key piece here is to know your part in the bigger structure. You may not be the quarterback, but your job might be the one that clears that path for him to score goals. That's a critical job. It's just behind the scenes. Like a stage manager. Or an editor. If you're not the coach, then be open to the feedback he or she gives you. The coach giving you feedback is in his or her role. Your role is to receive it.

TELL YOUR STORY

What does it mean to be "coachable" in your profession? Are you seeking out feedback from others you trust?

How do you respond when someone gives you feedback? How do you respond when you are challenged in conversation? Do you immediately reply, or do you take the feedback and think about it for a while? Do you typically react with more questions or firm answers? You probably respond differently to a partner than a peer at work. Consider those differences.

As you move through the day, notice situations where you did not get the outcome you wanted. Take the energy you might ordinarily have given to feeling frustrated, and use it to learn and incorporate new data. What approach would have a better outcome next time?

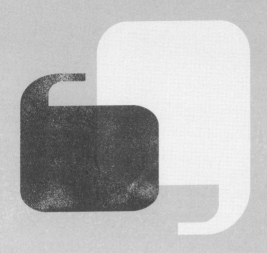

There are so many ways to look at the world. Why not appreciate a new angle?

Are you the same person from space to space?

As a person of color, I knew I would have to adapt a different cultural sensibility when I entered the academic arena. But I also knew I did not want to be disloyal to my community. The ivory tower prowess demanded something of me that called my integrity into question. I knew I could not become something my grandmother wouldn't recognize. I knew I could not become something my mother wouldn't recognize. How could I hold true to who I was, who my family helped develop, when I was also being told, "That doesn't fly here. You're not going to be successful if you hold on to that stuff"? This dilemma brought forth the idea of double-consciousness, described by W. E. B. DuBois in *The Souls of Black Folk*, an internal conflict of being Black in a country that centers whiteness. I carried a burden of doubleness—I was participating in the white culture of academia while being oppressed by that culture.

I reframed my time at the university as a quest. *I will go into the ivory tower. I will attain the secrets held there, and I will translate them into something that can meaningfully impact my community.* It took me five and a half years to get my PhD, while I saw white colleagues, not struggling with that double-consciousness, finish in four and a half years. Pushing back against the system cost me time. But that was me holding my integrity. I was learning the lingo, assuming the Westernized structures of presenting my ideas, and advancing through the process—all the while making sure I was the person my family would recognize when I emerged.

Unpacking racialized systems and structures in American society was crucial to my research, but folks on my dissertation committee said they didn't believe my field of study was relevant or meaningful. I knew there was no way I could discuss therapy and intervention outside the lens and context of race. That context was a cornerstone of my work. I ended up having to change my committee. That took time and disrupted the trajectory of my process, but it was necessary for remaining the same person in that space that I am everywhere else.

At this time I was studying Internal Family Systems therapy. In that framework, we imagine each individual containing a family of people. There's Corey as the father, Corey as the son, Corey as the husband, the coach, the therapist, the friend. We all have different ways of presenting ourselves, different versions of ourselves. Presenting a different part of yourself doesn't mean you're a liar; it means you're adaptable. It may also mean you're protecting yourself. It may be appropriate! When I attended university, I had to show up as Corey the student. That version of me may have presented a little bit differently than I would to my wife or my kids, but at my core, I held on to the exact same person underneath. I didn't lose the core Corey. I couldn't.

You see, you need to know the central *you* who is present in all the roles you play. We have to know who we are, at our core, to be able to do the rest of our work. The core person has to decide who will lead in any situation. When the core person doesn't decide who shows up, we can become fragmented. If we don't know who we are and we are at the mercy of whatever parts of us decide to show up, we may start to feel inauthentic or distant from how we present in certain spaces.

If you don't know who you are at your core, you might start to compromise key values or belief systems. It doesn't feel good. This is challenging for everyone, but if you're a person of color or in a minority group, you may be particularly challenged with this question. You've likely been asked to shed parts of you that are core to who you are. A word of wisdom—it's not worth it.

Adapt, listen, and learn—take on new roles and explore new ways of being—but never shed the core version of yourself for the comfort of others.

TELL YOUR STORY

What are the roles you play in various spaces in your life? Write a character description for each one. How does this person speak? How does this person hold himself or herself? How does that person thrive and struggle? Are any key words present across all your descriptions? These words may lead you to identifying your essence, your core.

Have you ever been in a space that challenged your integrity, just by the very fact of you being there? What are some ways you can maintain integrity in different spaces?

Have you ever had to push back against an institutionalized authority? What was your experience? How did you stay strong in that effort? What resources did you draw on?

What spaces make you the most uncomfortable, where you feel least like yourself? Throughout the week, if you notice yourself adopting a role that doesn't feel genuine, take note of it. Why do you think you adopted that role? What could you do differently next time?

Do you trust that the moment will unfold the way it's supposed to?

Too often people say we have to make the right choice. Rather, I think, like my mom taught me, we have to make the choice right. As I mentioned earlier, she first gave me this advice when I went off to undergrad at Long Beach, but I've carried this wisdom with me through every major life change I've ever made. I meet so many people—particularly young people—who are anxious about if they've made the right choices in life. They doubt and react and second-guess themselves trying to find some elusive "right" choice that will unlock their happiness, but here's the secret—you can't. The "right" choice doesn't exist.

All that exists is you and the present moment. Once you become aware of your genius and values—the one you're passionate about—everything you do should connect to that. And here's the fun part, kind of a curveball toward the end of the book. Sometimes you'll need to stand still. That doesn't mean you're not working hard, staying passionate and driven, and looking forward to the next goal, but you're not forcing things that don't fit. You're going to trust your sensibilities. Trust that your hard work will lead you where you need to go.

Sometimes we don't need to make a decision. Sometimes being still is the work. Being patient. Letting things unfold. I'm not asking you to approach the world the same way I do, but I'm hoping we can all find more moments to be in the moment. Granny Georgie told me that you need to develop a high level of awareness with self and, out of that, you can trust what unfolds. Watch. Pay attention. We have everything we need for the moment that's coming. Do you trust that you are already living in the abundance of what you need to be the best version of yourself?

For the past few years, I have been giving presentations at major universities around the country. I'm often asked to send a PowerPoint. I know a lot of people like to have a clear agenda. *Here's what we will talk about first. And here's what we will talk about next,* they tell the audience with their slides. They want measures. They want safeguards against going off topic. They're often distrustful of a fluid space. I, on the other hand, love the fluid space. I'd rather the agenda be developed in the moment through the conversation, laughter, genuine emotion, curiosity.

When I go in and do a more conversational presentation, letting myself feel my way in the moment, like I used to on the football field, I usually get a good response. "Doc, that was powerful," the people coordinating the presentation tell me. "Now I understand what you mean about not having all these parameters and borders." I let the conversation move in whatever direction it goes, using the moment, building on the momentum of the conversation. I trust the process to unfold. I can't tell you exactly what that will look like ahead of time. It's alive. If someone asks me a question I didn't expect, that's an opportunity to practice vulnerability. If someone in the audience is confused, that's an opportunity for me to clarify my own thinking. As much as I'm eager to share, I'm really just as eager to learn.

Think of talking to a friend. You don't say, "What are we going to talk about first? When will that end? And what will we talk about next?" We let the conversation unfold with, if we're lucky, laughter, genuine emotion, and curiosity. Why don't we apply that framework to other spaces?

In therapy I don't need to plan each step of the session. I may hold some expertise, but each of us is an expert in our own lives. The only expert in your life is you. Why would I try to impose my expertise on you? That's why I'm asking you so many questions. I will hear themes and see patterns. I'll pull at them and ask more questions. The story and the moment have everything that we need. We just need to let them unfold.

TELL YOUR STORY

In what areas of your life is it difficult to relinquish control? Is it harder for you to relinquish control in some areas of life more than others?

Identify a space where you don't want to relinquish control. What makes you nervous about trusting the moment to unfold? What's the very worst thing that could happen? Alternatively, what would you gain if you took your hands off?

Think about the people around you. Do you trust them? Can they share part of your burden? And conversely, are you willing to let them share part of your success?

Make a list of decisions you made in the last year, some big and some small. Take each decision you listed—even if you feel overall it wasn't the best decision for you—and list five ways that it turned out to be "right." Were there any moments of unexpected goodness that came to you? A new partner? A new job or skill? Did you clarify some nonnegotiables?

Does your life have movement?

Let's say someone takes poison and pours it into a pond. If you go back and test the water, the poison is still there. If someone puts poison in a river, on the other hand, when they test the water they'll find the poison is gone. The river is continuously flowing. That's not a strike on ponds; they're static. That's their role. But it's not our role to be static.

We must be rivers. We must have movement. I don't mean you need to move to another country. And you certainly don't need to be frenetic, filling up your days and running from one place to the next. But metaphorically and psychologically, you must stay fertile, present, and open to life's inevitable changes. Movement gives clarity. Movement gives moments of discovery. Let us all move toward being rivers, not ponds. In perpetual motion, never ceasing, never ending. Let's continuously regenerate. Let's go with the flow and be fluid.

You know by now that I like to look at our lives from the perspective of stories. Stories consist of forward motion. As the author of your own story, you must make meaningful decisions and act on them. I now live in a world largely comprised of language. I love the metaphor of the river and love using metaphors to express the inexpressible. The language I speak now is far from the physical language that I spoke for the first three decades of my life. But I know actions are still the basis for how we move forward and how we determine if we're living according to our values and our purpose. Sports trained me to stay present and to always maintain a sense of movement within myself—even in still moments. You can strategize about who runs where and who catches what, but all the talk, the sketches, and the pep talks mean little until you're out on the field or the court. You have to be alive to the moment, in every cell of your being, if you want to stay on your feet.

I mentioned this bit of advice from my dad earlier in the book. He used to say, "Your actions speak so loudly, I can't hear your words." Advice for writers and advice for life. Show me, don't tell me. Out on the field or court of your life, it's your actions that matter.

After my dad died, the world just kept rushing along, as if he were never here. As if his death didn't matter. People were going to school, playing basketball, going on dates. They were laughing. *How were they laughing?* I was stuck in a warp of my grief. I just lost one of the most meaningful people ever in my life. I remember thinking *The world doesn't notice when something like this happens. Am I lost in this? Am I missing something?*

I tried to keep up appearances, but my grief held me stagnant underneath, with a facade of movement, of moving on. *On to the next thing. Come along. Let's go.* No one was actually helping me move in a genuine way that processed the loss of my dad, helped me integrate his memory, and truly move forward. My life was motion without forward movement. It took me a few decades and becoming a father myself to figure out what it really meant to integrate the rush of life with my inner flow.

And I do believe you can go with the flow and end up where you want to be. If you have a dream and a passion and you outwork those around you, you will not have to search for success. It will find you. It will seek you out. It will almost attack you.

In childhood my grandmother had given me that vote of confidence, yet more than two decades later, I didn't think I could pursue an intellectual path. In my mind, I had failed academically. If I jumped back into that world, I would fall flat on my face. But that's not what happened. I reached out to professors. I started to do research. I figured out an approach and even started to like statistics. As I mentioned earlier, I had a mentor who was willing to push me forward with my writing. That meant revising and redoing and rewriting and practice,

practice, practice. Tear it up, do it again. Practice. I'd always been that discerning person my grandmother recognized. But it was the practice, the forward motion, saying goodbye to the old version of myself, showing up for the academic work the way I'd shown up on the field—that got me from a nervous, curious student to a therapist who gets to live my days filled with ideas. With observation. With discernment.

With conversation.

Playing football throughout high school and college taught me a lot about staying in the moment and going with the flow. I studied the plays, had all the patterns down pat. But sometimes the play goes sideways—the river splits—and every second you have to adjust, recalibrate, choose, act. That's when all the practice, all the introspection, all the truth telling by the coaches had better be deep in your gut. Because sometimes on the field, as in life, the moment is now.

And the river keeps rushing along.

TELL YOUR STORY

What would it look like to be more flexible and fluid today? Think of three things you could do that would embody "going with the flow." Do you want to give any of them a try?

Do any areas of your life feel stagnant, like ponds? Maybe it's an unexplored hobby. A friendship that no longer fits. A dream of learning to paint that's always relegated to the realm of "someday." List out these "ponds" and pick one that you want to explore more fully.

Look back over the work you've done in this book. What elements can serve as tributaries for your river? Maybe it's allowing yourself to imagine your future. Maybe it's discovering your essence. Maybe it's learning to put yourself first or getting clarity on your values. Pick two or three areas that stand out and give yourself space to consider how they can help direct you toward a life with greater movement.

Grace

Through your journey in this book, I hope you've realized that how you are doing depends a lot on you and the actions you take in the story you're telling. You can take those actions intentionally. You can be curious when things aren't going the way you think they should or when others provide feedback that might be hard to hear. You have agency. That makes you powerful. That also makes you vulnerable.

Urie Bronfenbrenner was a psychologist born in Moscow in 1917, and he moved to the United States as a young child. His ecological systems theory focused on the complex and inter-active system dynamics that shape a child's development. One of the ideas in this theory always stood out to me. It's the idea of ecotones as a kind of borderland where two spaces meet and partially overlap. Think of a city meeting the first-rung suburb; you have an ecotone. It's not fully urban. It's not fully suburban. You can watch a Twins baseball game, then on your way out of the stadium you might see a deer dashing into the woods. Or perhaps it's easier to picture a tidal area of a seashore, with its rich diversity of species.

The ecotone can refer to sociocultural, interpersonal, and introspective spaces as well. They're the in-between spaces where you get the greatest variety. With the awareness you're gaining and the curiosity you're practicing, you are at a kind of ecotone now—a fertile, in-between place of great variety. I hope you can enjoy that multiplicity and embrace the unknown.

I know it can be frightening. I've talked throughout the book about the playground. I asked you to invite me into it. But I've also acknowledged that not all our work is fun. Not all of it is swinging from the monkey bars.

My mom was a lab technician, and my dad had been a veteran. When I was a child, we had an enormous machine in our living room. The Veterans Administration purchased it for us and trained my mother. Three times a week my mom would hook my dad up to that machine for kidney dialysis. He had two kidney transplants. They worked for a while, and then his body began to reject them. This was huge, but nobody was discussing it. Nobody looked at me and said, "How are you doing? What's your sense? How are you dealing with this?" I felt like I didn't have anyone. But I got it. I caught the lesson. I guess we don't talk about this. We just move on.

When Dad passed out, I would hold his head upside down so the blood would rush back to his brain. As a nine-year-old child, I held Dad's head on a regular basis. Those scenes, I believe, are the primal root of a fear I carried with me into adulthood. "I'm gonna lose him," that young Corey said to himself about his father. "You're not gonna be around, Dad. I'm scared that you're not gonna be around." No one seemed to recognize that this nine-year-old boy was struggling. The same was true after my dad died. I deeply wanted someone to say something to me. To say, "How are you doing?" But they didn't have the words.

Now my life's work is trying to help people find the words they need. To ask them how they're doing. And to listen when they tell me.

I've done a hell of a lot of my own therapy. I've trusted other therapists to guide me, and I've worked on myself. When I started to do this work, I had to confront the loss of my father and the pain that child faced. Having lost my dad, how do I keep his legacy alive? How do I talk to my boys about who he was to me? I had sons at about the same age as my dad was when he had kids. How I'm fathering them is related to how he fathered me. This work brought me to the moment where I looked at that nine-year-old Corey and told him, "You don't have to be scared."

Eight months ago from the time of writing this, my sister passed away. You might remember she was the reason I chose to go to Long Beach State for college, because she lived in Southern California. When it was time for her to leave this world, my sister knew I knew she was leaving. We tend not to talk about this kind of thing. I went through my father's body failing with no one saying a word. But this time I was going to change the narrative. I wasn't going to be that scared boy with no one to talk to.

I told my sister, Sharon, "I want you to know a few things about who you've been to me." I told her she'd live on through stories I'd tell my sons. I would continue to bring forth her name. I was vulnerable in those moments, but they freed me. Or I should say *"And* they freed me." *Both/and,* one of my favorite phrases. We know vulnerability releases us into freedom. Sharon wasn't abandoning me, just like my father hadn't been abandoning me during childhood. Sharon wasn't going to disappear.

It was simply her turn to move on. Into the ecotone.

When we connect through open conversations, it makes us lighter. This is the root of therapy. Whenever I can, I bring levity to our conversations. Like I said in the entry about humor, if we can laugh, even in the toughest conversations, we know we're going to be all right. But there are times we can't laugh. There are times we have to dig way down into our pain. To fully heal, to truly grow, there's sometimes no getting around it.

In these months since Sharon has moved on, I get to have my sister around me continuously. It's a thing of beauty that came from the chaos and sadness of her death. In some ways, I'm closer to her now than I ever was at Long Beach State.

Maybe even more than I ever was in Arkansas City, Kansas, three miles up from the Oklahoma border, in the house next to my grandparents. She's always with me now.

I choose to move through life with a blanket of grace over me. If you saw your wife or child or roommate curled up asleep on the couch, would you take the blanket and cover them with it? I'm guessing it'd be the first thing you'd do. Will you do the same for yourself? Can you tell the truth, move to forgiveness with yourself, and produce a blanket of grace you can lay over yourself that will allow you to move forward? I hope this book is an opportunity to begin to do that work. I hope you can find happiness from loss, beauty from chaos and sadness. I hope you find communion.

I'm going to visualize you now. You're in a quiet room. Maybe the leaves on the trees outside the window have turned red and are starting to fall. You take a deep breath, grab hold of your pen, and keep writing the story of your life. You're embracing forward motion and the constant series of goodbyes that you know it requires.

Revel in your discoveries. Find the exciting possibilities inherent in dissonance resolving into harmony, and the process repeating again. As the tide goes in and out, you'll find a new rhythm in change, if you want to. But I don't want to push change on you. I am happy with awareness. With curiosity, truth telling, intentionality, and vulnerability setting you free. Change is up to you.

Sources

Barnett, Ronald and Norman Jackson, eds. *Ecologies for Learning and Practice: Emerging Ideas, Sightings, and Possibilities.* United Kingdom: Taylor & Francis, 2019.

DuBois, W. E .B. *The Souls of Black Folk.* New York: New American Library: 2012.

Markham, Laurie, David Epston, and David Marsten. *Narrative Therapy in Wonderland: Connecting with Children's Imaginative Know-How.* New York: W. W. Norton & Company, 2016.

Pittman, John P. "Double Consciousness." *Stanford Encyclopedia of Philosophy* (Summer 2016). https://plato.stanford.edu/archives /sum2016/entries/double-consciousness/.

Sartre, Jean-Paul. "Man Is Condemned to Be Free." From lecture, "Existentialism Is a Humanism." 1946. Translated by Philip Mairet, 1948. https://wmpeople.wm.edu/asset/index/cvance /sartre.

Sweezy, Martha and Richard C. Schwartz. *Internal Family Systems Therapy.* Second Edition. United States: Guilford Publications, 2019.

University of St. Augustine for Health Sciences. "How Laughter Can Relieve Stress + Ideas to Laugh it Off." *USAHS Blog.* November 2019. https://www.usa.edu/blog/how-laughter-can -relieve-stress/.

Notes

1. "How Many Cells Are in the Human Body? Fast Facts," Healthline.com, https://www.healthline.com/health/number-of-cells-in-body#human-cells.
2. *Merriam-Webster.com Dictionary*, s.v. "genius," Merriam-Webster, accessed November 16, 2021, https://www.merriam-webster.com/dictionary/genius.
3. One of the universities in the U.S. with the greatest amount of research activity.
4. Henry David Thoreau, *Walden* (New York: Penguin, 1999), 72. Originally published in 1854.

Acknowledgments

Relationships are the most important things I have discovered across my lifetime, so it is only fitting for me to spotlight just a few of the most impactful ones that have played a pivotal role in my existence. I realize that as I highlight many, I will also shadow some very important ones. I apologize in advance for not being able to recognize all who have impacted me in profound ways.

A heartfelt thank you to several people who helped create the journey you took in this book. First, thank you to my friend and acquisitions editor, Danielle Peterson. DP, you understood my quirky way of being from the outset and stood by my side throughout the book-writing endeavor! I am forever indebted!

To Michael Aulisio, the VP/Publisher of Harper Celebrate, thank you for your persistence and support, and most of all, thank you for believing in me and having a clear vision for the creation of this book.

To Rachel Federman, my partner in writing *How Am I Doing?*, I am so thankful for the hours you dedicated to this project. You have truly become a dear friend.

To my literary agent, Heidi Krupp, thanks for being the best in the business, and even more, thank you for understanding and supporting me through this new venture. You have been rock solid, and I am deeply appreciative for all that you have done for me.

Cindy Mori is much more than a manager to me. As my sister-in-love, friend, business partner, and visionary, it is clear to me that there would be no How Am I Doing? were it not for your patience, thoughtfulness, and candor. Thank you simply for being you! I can't wait to see what is next for us!

I must give a special thanks to Coach Dwane Casey of the Detroit Pistons and his wife, Brenda. Coach, I am deeply appreciative to you for providing me the opportunity to join this first-class organization, and how you and Brenda have invited me into your world and treated me as part of your family.

To my wife, Carrie, and "suns," Izaiah, Zach, and Azrie, there are literally no words that can express my love and gratitude for each of you! Carrie, you saw in me so much potential from the moment we met. You have been and continue to be the love of my life, my partner, and my confidant. Without your love and support, none of this would have been possible! Izaiah, thank you for teaching me what unconditional love is and what it means to be a genuine human! Zach, your hard work and dedication have become a cornerstone to how I see and move in this world! Azrie, watching you grow into a young man of unwavering substance and discernment has been an undeniable pleasure. This Yeager family unit has become the foundation of all that is me! I will forever be in debt to you each individually, and more importantly, collectively. It's difficult to express in words the ways that you've impacted me, but I hope to demonstrate my gratitude each and every day in my relationships with you.

Growing up, I had so many influential people that molded me into who I am today and whose legacies live on in these pages. Thank you to my mama, Beverly Yeager. You are the best mom a kid could have! Although I had him for only fifteen short years, my father, Harlan Percy Yeager, taught me what it was to be a man of love and integrity. Granny and Papa, thank you for taking the time to love and guide me through some tough times. To my siblings, Uriah and Sharon, a little brother could not have been as fortunate as I was to have you two as guideposts! Sharon, you may not any longer be with us physically, but you are clearly with me in spirit. Thank you to my nephew JD Dubois, for teaching me so much about you and about myself! Thank you to my mentors Dr. Bill Doherty and Dr. Jim Nelson, and to my friends like Ty and Kirra Abington, who have been invaluable to my journey. Friends that came into my life over the recent years, like Michael Walker and Shawn Shipman, have helped me understand that real dawgs can be found throughout our lives. Although we lost you far too early, Nash and Matt Gee, your friendships live on in my memory forever.

Finally, I am thankful for the struggles, mishaps, and stumbles across my lifetime. Those very struggles taught me so much about myself. I hope to forever be a river, moving and regenerating my existence. Onward, with gratitude.

About the Author

Best known for his appearance on Prince Harry and Oprah's *The Me You Can't See* on Apple TV+, Dr. Corey Yeager is a licensed marriage and family therapist at the doctoral level, focusing primarily on serving the African American community. His research emphasis centers on better understanding the plight of African American relationships. In his current role as the psychotherapist for the Detroit Pistons, Dr. Yeager is merging his two passions, athletics and therapy. He currently resides in Minneapolis, Minnesota, with his wife, Carrie, and four sons, Izaiah, Zach, Azrie, and Terrance.